Praise for *The Power of Stillness* by Tobin Blake

"A helpful book on simplifying the stepping-stones to stilling the mind."
— **Gerald G. Jampolsky, MD**, author of *Love Is Letting Go of Fear*

"I love this book. It is clear, original, interesting, welcoming, and above all, helpful. I can't imagine anyone who would not benefit from reading even a small part of it. I especially like the deeper understanding Blake brings to the subject of prayer within a book on meditation."
— **Hugh Prather**, author of
How to Live in the World and Still Be Happy

"This wise book grounds the reader in the great meditative traditions while offering a clear framework for practicing in today's busy world. Tobin Blake does more than just point out the path to serenity; he is a knowledgeable guide to the points of interest and the pitfalls along the way."
— **Patricia Monaghan**, coauthor of *Meditation: The Complete Guide*
and *Encyclopedia of Goddesses and Heroines*

"There is a revelation in stillness; it opens us to the Divine, and expands our awareness. Meditation is really an open secret and the most precious of spiritual practices. Tobin Blake understands the meaning of stillness and has learned it through his own meditation experience. As practical as it is profound, *The Power of Stillness* is an effective evocation of the desire to sit, to just be."
— **Wayne Teasdale**, author of *The Mystic Heart*

Praise for *Everyday Meditation* by Tobin Blake

"This lovely book is a quiet encouragement to the deep peace and healing that meditation brings. It is what each of us — and the whole world — needs now; and the loving spirit in which it is written is, clearly, a gift of meditation. Read it and feel joy; practice it, and be transformed."
— **Daphne Rose Kingma**, author of
The Ten Things to Do When Your Life Falls Apart
and *The Future of Love*

"Tobin Blake's *Everyday Meditation* guides you gently into the stream of a healing and life-enhancing meditation practice. The daily practices fit with our busy lives and are never overwhelming but designed to build confidence and skill one day at a time. A valuable hands-on guide for beginners as well as long-time meditators seeking a variety of techniques."

— **Donald Altman**, author of *One-Minute Mindfulness*
and *The Mindfulness Code*

the healing
of jordan young

Also by Tobin Blake

Everyday Meditation

The Power of Stillness

the healing of jordan young

A 21ST-CENTURY SPIRITUAL GUIDE TO HEALTH AND HEALING

Tobin Blake

FOREWORD BY DR. BERNIE S. SIEGEL

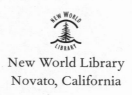

New World Library
Novato, California

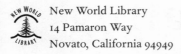 New World Library
14 Pamaron Way
Novato, California 94949

The material in this book is intended for education. It is not meant to take the place of diagnosis and treatment by a qualified medical practitioner or therapist. No expressed or implied guarantee of the effects of the use of the recommendations can be given nor liability taken. Some names have been changed to protect the privacy of individuals.

Text design by Tona Pearce Myers

Library of Congress Cataloging-in-Publication Data is available.

First printing, November 2015
ISBN 978-1-60868-354-3
Printed in Canada on 100% postconsumer-waste recycled paper

 New World Library is proud to be a Gold Certified Environmentally Responsible Publisher. Publisher certification awarded by Green Press Initiative. www.greenpressinitiative.org

10   9   8   7   6   5   4   3   2   1

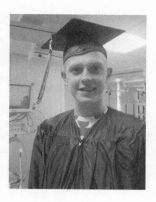

This book is dedicated with love to my daughter Brittany, who at the tender age of seventeen displayed uncommon courage, maturity, and sensitivity as she watched — and supported — Jordan, her high school sweetheart and first love, while he fought for his life. I'm not sure that I could have done the same when I was her age. Indeed, I am quite certain that I would have failed miserably by comparison. I have no doubt that Brittany is a soul destined for great things in this world. I love you, my dear daughter, and I am prouder of you than words could ever express.

Also, to the thousands of friends and family of patients facing similar battles around the world every day. Do not underestimate your role as caregivers and supporters of those who are struggling with fear and disease. Your love and companionship is a precious, healing elixir; apply liberally!

Contents

Foreword by Dr. Bernie S. Siegel   xi

Introduction: The Guy Who Survived   xix

Part One: Principles of Healing

Chapter One: Minding Your Mind   3

Chapter Two: The Seeds of Disease   15

Chapter Three: Mind Over Matter   37

Chapter Four: Into the Desert of Fear   55

Part Two: Special Principles of Healing

Chapter Five: The Patient Must Believe Healing Is Possible   67

Chapter Six: The Patient Must Want to Heal   75

Chapter Seven: New Hope: "Smart" Chemo and
Bone Marrow Transplants   95

Chapter Eight: The Patient Must Feel They Deserve to Heal   105

Part Three: Methods of Healing

Chapter Nine: Reprogramming the Waterfall of Thought   125
Chapter Ten: On a Wing and a Prayer   135
Chapter Eleven: A Guide to Meditation   143
Chapter Twelve: The Art of Visualization   165
Chapter Thirteen: The Intensive Care Unit   175
Chapter Fourteen: The Power of Prayer and Affirmations   179
Chapter Fifteen: "You Mean I'm Not Going to Make It?"   187
Chapter Sixteen: Laying Hands, Holding Presence,
    and Unity   195
Chapter Seventeen: The Mystery of the Melting Tumors   205
Chapter Eighteen: Support Networks and Spiritual
    Relationships   213
Chapter Nineteen: A String of "Co-Incidences"   223
Chapter Twenty: A Brief Guide for Friends, Family,
    and Healers   229

Epilogue: Jordan Lived!   243
Acknowledgments   247
Appendix: Principles of Healing and Special Principles
    of Healing   249
Endnotes   250
Recommended Reading   251
About the Author   253

Foreword

*F*or me, writing a foreword to this book was like writing a book about the book itself. In his introduction Tobin Blake states that he is not a doctor. Well, I am a doctor, though not your typical or average doctor because of my life and experience counseling and running cancer support groups for patients who, because of their qualities, have been my teachers for forty years. *The Healing of Jordan Young* is a true guide to health and healing. It is a unique story that contains vast amounts of wisdom. However, I find it sad that people have to keep discovering the wisdom through their own tragedies and then write a book about their experience, thinking they have something unique to share. I am saying this in the hope that you will take the time to read on, learn from the wisdom of others, and not require a disaster to become your teacher. It is very therapeutic to turn a curse into a blessing, but why not learn how to find the blessing in your life without requiring the curse? Our difficulties can lead us to heal, just as hunger can lead us to seek nourishment, but it is a lot healthier to create a life that is nourishing so we do not need to be driven and motivated by hunger and difficulties.

The body believes what the mind conceives and visualizes. It is a case of mind over matter, because what your heart and mind sense matters, and it creates our internal chemistry and environment. Over the years I have come to realize our potential for healing and that we can all learn from the success of others when we stop fearing failure, guilt, shame, and blame. I have heard many stories from people who are alive today because of self-induced healing, and their themes always have much in common. We can all learn from the success of others and believe in what we and they experience. I use the term "self-induced healing" because that is what is created when one makes the necessary changes. It is not a spontaneous remission from which there is nothing to learn. We all, including health professionals, need to learn from success and the truth and not wait until science believes, studies, and validates the truth.

In his novel *Cancer Ward*, Aleksandr Solzhenitsyn describes self-induced healing as a "rainbow-colored butterfly" fluttering out of the open book one of the men is reading from to the other patients, sharing with them that there are cases of self-induced healing and not recovery through treatment. That symbol says it all, the butterfly being the symbol of transformation and the rainbow the symbol of a life of order and emotional harmony. When people create that new life, their bodies respond to their internal chemistry, related to their now loving their lives and bodies. When we choose life, meaning a life that is life-enhancing for all of creation, amazing things happen. Tobin Blake and Jordan Young are examples we can all learn from.

Healing is not about fighting a war against an enemy or a disease. Doing that empowers the enemy. Healing is about finding peace and not attending antiwar rallies but attending peace rallies. Spirituality is a significant factor in turning a curse into a blessing.

When we are willing to ask ourselves what lessons we are to learn from our journey through hell, amazing things occur, and they are not coincidences but miracles created by the future we unconsciously prepared.

For us to find our truth, certain things must happen. First, we must live by our experience and not let our beliefs create a situation where we close our minds. Our Creator has given all living things an enormous potential for healing, surviving, and thriving. However, if we do not have self-love because of a life experience of abuse and rejection, our resulting self-destructive behavior will prevent us from achieving our potential. The path to healing starts with the symbolism of the still pond. It is only when our mind, like the water, is free of turbulence that we can see the true reflection and recognize that we are not ugly ducklings but swans. Then through meditation, imagery, prayer, faith, dreams, and inner voices, we can be guided by consciousness on the path to healing. The physical benefits that accompany it are not coincidences. As a physician, I know the power of patients' beliefs — and the benefits or problems they can create.

There is a survivor personality, a.k.a. immune-competent personality, and therapists are more aware of it than doctors are. Doctors are informed about disease but not educated about people, so they tend to treat the result and not the cause. We prescribe pills for a diagnosis without asking about what patients are experiencing and helping them to live between office visits. This should not be about blaming patients but showing them how their lives' conditions affect their health. I have sent articles about my experience to medical journals, only to have them returned as "interesting but inappropriate for our journal." When I sent the same articles to psychology journals, they were returned as "appropriate but not interesting." Doctors need to recognize each person as an entity and not treat only parts of the person but treat the whole person and their experience of life. We all need to learn from success and not toss it aside as spontaneous or miraculous. Doctors need to ask their patients, "Why didn't you die when I expected you to?"

I know innumerable people who accepted their mortality and went off to enjoy the last few months of their lives. When I realized I hadn't been invited to attend their funerals, I called to scold the families for ignoring me, only to have the people I thought had died answer the phone. "It was so beautiful here I forgot to die," one said. We now have studies showing that loneliness and laughter affect the genes that control immune function. So relationships, sense of purpose, lifestyle, and more affect our health and survival.

This book tells us that with love nothing is impossible, and I know from experience that is true. So love yourself and your life and accept that you are a child of God: made of the same stuff and capable of accomplishing amazing things. Life is a miracle, and you are a part of life.

If you grew up without love but with indifference, rejection, and abuse, you have your work cut out for you. So do not put this book down. Read it and let us reparent you and help you find your authenticity and potential for self-healing. You can abandon your past and move forward. Studies show that 98 percent of children who felt lonely and unloved experience a major illness by middle age, while only 24 percent of those who felt loved as children experience a major illness by middle age. How can we save ourselves?

Actors' immune functioning is improved when they act in comedies and decreased in tragedies, while their stress hormone levels are lowered in comedies and elevated in tragedies. We are all actors given a lifetime to rehearse and practice, so start acting as if you were the person you want to be, and let Jordan and Tobin be your life coaches and directors as you perform.

Studies reveal that when you incorporate gratitude and meditation into your daily routine, your telomeres lengthen. So in a sense you are growing younger because of your lifestyle and mental state. Also, cancer patients who laugh several times a day for no reason and practice gratitude and meditation daily have better survival statistics. However, we are healed not only by what we do but also by what we think and believe. As I said, the body believes what the mind visualizes as the truth. So our thoughts and *wordswordswords* can become *swordswordswords* that can either kill or cure depending upon how one uses them. When doctors treat people in the same way that one would renovate a house, meaning different parts require different specialists, the patients' unity and wholeness are not treated, and what results is not repair or healing but just mechanical changes.

When we have faith in those treating us and believe in the treatment we are receiving, we respond in a positive way. I know of cases where patients were not receiving chemotherapy or radiation due to equipment repair mistakes and medical errors, but the doctors did not realize it for many weeks. Why? Because the patients experienced side effects and their tumors shrunk. The patients weren't being treated but thought they were, and their bodies acted as if they were being treated, thus confusing the doctors — but also showing them the power of the mind. I have learned we can deceive people into health, too, with our words and their beliefs.

The opposite of love is indifference and rejection, not fear or hate. Love heals and empowers, but we have to let the love in. And if we do not induce healing, we must not judge ourselves as failures or think it means we didn't love enough. Our potential is there for us, and we can become responsible participants rather than submissive sufferers. Guilt, shame, and blame can be imposed by authority figures and religions that claim that our disease is punishment, but, remember, disease is a loss of health, and this book has been written to empower you and help you find what you have lost. If you can't find your car keys, you don't assume God wants you to walk home. So when you lose your health, look for it and get others to help you. Hope is never false, and when a chemotherapy program with four drugs beginning with the letters E, P, O and H was called the EPOH Protocol and was tested, 25 percent of patients did well. One doctor decided to reverse the letters and give the HOPE Protocol, and 75 percent of his patients responded positively. And I don't make up any of the stories I tell.

As quantum physicists tell us, desire and intention alter the physical world, causing things to occur that would not normally occur if they were not desired. So read on, and whatever your life's challenge is, give it your best shot. You can burst the dam that restricts and blocks the flow of your life and let the released energy move you forward. One way of helping yourself heal is to ask yourself what words describe what it is like to experience cancer or whatever problem you are living with. Think about whether the negative words you come up with fit other problems that exist in your life. Eliminate those things and help yourself heal your life and find your rainbow. If you come up with a new beginning or wake-up call, you are on the right track.

Sharing your wounds can also help you heal. We are all wounded, so be honest with the people close to you and help one another to heal. The wounded soldier serves and helps us all. A woman from North Carolina with leukemia was told she had two months to live and little hope from any chemotherapy. She came to see me because one of her relatives knew of my work. I sat on her bed, shared with her, and hugged her. I asked my oncologist friend, who was aware of my "crazy patients," to come and see her. He said he agreed with her doctor but knew my patients and would give her hope. In two months she was in complete remission and went home to drive her doctor nuts. She told her cousin that when I'd sat on her bed and hugged her, she knew she would get well.

Life is a school, and we must understand that if the world were perfect, it would have no meaning. We are all here to live and learn, and personally I think our mortality is our greatest teacher and can induce us to define and live what I call our "chocolate ice cream" — to live in a way that makes us happy. In many ways I believe death is a commencement, too. However, while attending the school of life, remember that the energy of creation is available to all of us. Health professionals, healers, and family can all be the battery cables that help direct the healing energy into our bodies, recharge our batteries, and give us the power to heal.

Stop judging, and keep learning from your difficult journey. Spiritual flat tires happen. What are spiritual flat tires? The ones that make you miss a plane that you later learn crashed after takeoff. Stop judging and just be. As my mom used to say, "God is redirecting you. Something good will come of this."

Prayers are always answered but not always in the way we desire. When you are not capable of using the pain as a labor pain of self-birth, God will show up to assist you. But when it is time for you to step up and use the labor pains to give birth to a new and authentic self, God steps back so you can experience healthy growth and rebirth yourself. Remember, we and God are made of the same stuff, and when you get to Heaven and they ask how you want to be introduced to God, the right answers are "Tell God his child is here," or "Tell God It's me," or "Tell God His replacement is here." (The last answer actually came from a high school student I was talking to.)

My body is the gift I was given so I could attend and experience the school of life, help raise my level of consciousness, and help create a healthier future for us all — one in which we each have a reverence for all life. We are all family and the same color inside. Death is not a failure, so trying not to die is not the issue; living is. Someday when you get tired of your body, it is okay to turn off the life switch and become, as William Saroyan wrote, "dreamless, unalive perfect." I have seen my loved ones die laughing as we shared stories of their life and love while letting them go, free of guilt and feelings of failure, when their bodies were no longer a gift but were painful burdens. And as my ninety-seven-year-old father-in-law, who was quadriplegic because of a fall, said when asked for advice for seniors, "Tell them to just fall up." And he did just that when he was tired of life.

For me, healing and curing are two distinct entities. There are many people who are cured of an illness by their treatment but do not live healed lives, versus someone like Helen Keller, whom I consider to be healed and my teacher even though her physical disability was incurable. So being physically cured of disease and being healed are two separate things, and I seek out the healed to be my life coaches, knowing that when I heal my life I derive physical benefits, too. So become a love warrior: let love be your weapon of choice in all conflicts. And know that the only thing truer than the truth is a story.

After reading this enlightening book, ask yourself what you believe about healing and curing: Was Jordan healed and cured by his belief or by his treatment?

— Dr. Bernie S. Siegel, bestselling author of
The Art of Healing and *Love, Medicine & Miracles*

INTRODUCTION

The Guy Who Survived

W hat you are about to read is a true story. We've all heard versions of it: A guy gets diagnosed with incurable cancer, and his doctors give him only months to live. The family gathers, praying for a miracle while bracing for the worst, yet despite the odds, the guy survives. How does it happen? Is it just fate? Biological roulette? Stellar health care? The luck of the draw?

By the time I met Jordan Young, I had been studying meditation, healing, and the mind-body connection for over twenty years. When Jordan became ill, I knew it was no mere coincidence that we had become acquainted. It was what I call a "co-incidence," which is when two or more seemingly separate paths, people, or events are drawn together — not by chance — but by some invisible Cosmic thread that defies human comprehension. In short, I knew I had been put there in order to help Jordan heal, and it was a path I felt divinely guided to follow. I could not turn away.

Jordan came into my life through my daughter Brittany. The two were high school sweethearts, and they were thoroughly inseparable. Brittany and Jordan had been dating for two years by the time he was diagnosed with an aggressive form of lymphoma (cancer of the lymphatic system), which easily defeated every attempt to control it. By this time, Jordan had become a part of our family, and we all loved him. On a personal level, watching him fight to survive was one of the most heart-wrenching experiences of my life, and though I could not know it then, our journey together would transform the way I view sickness and healing forever.

Near the end of that spring, only months after his diagnosis, every available treatment option had failed, and Jordan rapidly began deteriorating. On June 11, 2012, mere days before he was set to graduate from high school, Jordan was airlifted by plane 175 miles from home and admitted to the intensive care unit of Oregon Health & Science University Hospital in Portland, which is one of the top research and treatment facilities in the Pacific Northwest. An MRI revealed that his lungs were choked with tumors, and he was actively suffocating. Doctors also discovered that the disease had infiltrated his liver, but strangely — relatively speaking — this seemed an insignificant detail compared to the fatal event that was unfolding inside his lungs.

They put Jordan on oxygen and dosed him with chemo, but the medical treatment at this point was more an effort to make him comfortable and slow his spiraling decline than to save his life. It was far too late for radiation, and chemotherapy had already failed three times in a row; it was not expected to magically begin working now.

The classic phrase "three strikes and you're out" comes to mind. Apparently the concept works the same in medicine as it does in baseball, though the stakes of this game were far higher — life or death.

Medicine has advanced a long way since the days of witch doctors and virgin sacrifices, but today's physicians still do not understand why one patient may recover when another does not, even when they suffer from identical illnesses and share similar medical profiles. In spite of all we have learned, when it comes to healing, it seems there are still more mysteries than known facts. One critical component we are beginning to understand for certain, however, is that a patient's thoughts, attitudes, emotions, and beliefs have an enormous impact on the healing process and on whether a given patient will recover from a given disease.

I was little more than a kid when I first heard about a supposedly "unexplained" healing. It was something I read about in a psychology textbook (that's not as strange as it may sound; my father was a psychologist, now retired, and I grew up surrounded by books about the subject). The story went something like this: A man developed untreatable cancer, and he decided he wanted to spend the last months of his life doing the thing he loved most, which happened to be *laughing*. So the guy spent the precious months following his diagnosis watching a barrage of his favorite, funny television shows and movies from his past, investing hour after hour engaged in the pursuit of pure joy.

The story ends happily, of course, with the guy making a full recovery and going on to share his incredible tale with the world. Inexplicably, he had laughed his cancer into remission.

Or so the story goes. Looking back, I do not know if this particular case is true, a fabrication, or somewhere in between, but it does not really matter. There are many examples of unexplained healings, and plenty of them have been documented. It is not the purpose of this book to examine such healings in order to prove that they were of spiritual, psychical, or miraculous origin. In fact, this book is not particularly concerned with "proving" anything, including in regards to Jordan's case. Rather, it is a simple book with a humble aim: to show how one boy's astonishing story of healing can inspire us all.

Whether you are a patient, someone who loves a patient, or just a person who treasures his or her health and wants to remain well, this book is set up to do much more than relate one person's journey through illness and healing. It will give you real tools you can use to stay healthy or, when the balance of health shifts toward disease, to stimulate the healing process — no matter what the distress, whether physical, mental, or spiritual. All are really the same when properly understood. We will be exploring a variety of spiritual healing principles and practices, some ancient, others contemporary, which you can implement in your life from the privacy of your own home, at no cost, beginning immediately.

The healing system derives from a blend of strategies based on some of the most powerful teachings I have ever encountered, along with my own experience. A great many healers have influenced the system, but if there has been one major influence, it has come from *A Course in Miracles*, one of the most remarkable teachings on healing ever recorded. The material presented here represents the best of what I've found over two decades' worth of study, meditation, and experience as a spiritual teacher. None of it is complicated, and the techniques require only a little time and effort to be effective.

The book consists of three primary parts: "Principles of Healing," "Special Principles of Healing," and "Methods of Healing," a few of which include meditation, visualization, focused prayer, and affirmations. The Principles of Healing are primarily theoretical in focus and content; however, these lessons represent the essential basis for the healing process. This section is broken down into seven primary principles in order to make it easier to assimilate and study the material. It is not that *seven* is a magic number. These same basic concepts could, perhaps, be condensed into fewer principles or, conversely, expanded into more. In this case, seven will serve our purpose in sufficient detail. The Special Principles of Healing in part 2 detail the essential psychological conditions that the patient must meet in order for healing to occur. Together with the primary Principles of Healing, these teachings form the backbone of the presented healing system. (For reference, a detailed list of all the principles is included in the appendix.)

This book is not meant to be a passive read; it is a healing device, intended to provide you with the knowledge and essential techniques, as well as the energy, you need in order to recover, to assist others in healing, or to live the healthiest life possible. During the course of writing it, I have attempted to ground myself in the present moment as much as possible and allow the Higher Intelligence of the universe — whatever you prefer to call that Intelligence, whether Source, God, Spirit, something else, or nothing at all — to work through me. This is meant to infuse the book with a background of natural healing energy, which you will absorb as you read along. This may sound like metaphysical nonsense, but I assure you nothing could be further from the truth. The universe we live in is composed of energy, including all forms of communication. Try to remain as quiet and present as possible while reading, and sense this energy. There is a spaciousness that can be felt in the present moment, which most of us are unaware of because we are constantly thinking of the past or projecting our thoughts into the future. Yet, as we will explore, all lasting healing originates in the present, as does all authentic joy.

It is best to consider healing, as well as the study of this material, as a journey and not a destination. This journey is an ongoing learning process that ideally should continue throughout your lifetime. I have by no means mastered it myself. Although I teach meditation and healing through spiritual awakening, ultimately I am still a student of Spirit, as are all of us who inhabit the earth, or what I call *Earth School*. We are all here to learn the same curriculum, which is the curriculum of awakening, and I have come to understand that all healing actually derives from awakening because awakening *is* the ultimate healing. What this means is, the form of the disease does not really matter; the cure for all distress is awakening.

Some of the material in the book may seem impossible, and some too simple to be true. I urge you to set your judgment aside and approach it with an open mind. Remember that judgment, in any form, will limit your perspective, and by doing so, it will reduce your options. That is to say, it will dictate what is possible and what is not possible — for *you*. Belief is a powerful force, as we will soon explore. Therefore it is wise to choose your beliefs with care. In general, when it comes to healing, you want *more options*, not fewer; you want a broader, more open mind, not a narrower one.

This is not to suggest that you *must* believe everything you are about to read in order to heal or stay healthy. I am merely inviting you to consider the possibilities and open your mind to a new understanding of health, where it comes from, how it is maintained, and how we can recover when we do get sick. If an idea doesn't make sense to you at first, try not to dismiss it. Perhaps it will become more meaningful to you as you proceed.

I am not a doctor. The information in this book is for educational use only. It is not intended to diagnose or treat any medical or psychiatric condition, nor replace treatment by a licensed physician or mental healthcare professional. If you are sick, go see a doctor...*please*. Then read this book! The healing system presented is meant as a *supplement* to modern medical and psychiatric care, and it will be most effective, for most patients, when applied in tandem with qualified, modern treatments.

While I have made every effort to provide accurate medical information when discussing Jordan's case, many of the medications and procedures he received were complicated and are difficult to describe without cluttering the text with laborious technical details. Rather than taking this route, I decided to keep things simple for the sake of clarity. Hence, the sections of the book that discuss the medical aspects of Jordan's journey are not designed to provide detailed medical guidance. They offer basic information meant to help the reader understand Jordan's struggles and, in general terms, how his treatments did their respective jobs.

One other complicating factor in relating Jordan's story involved the emotional turbulence and ensuing confusion that occurred during his illness — which everyone involved experienced to some degree — along with the fact that Jordan's doctors were forced to make complex decisions rapidly. This caused a significant challenge when, years later, I began piecing his journey back together for this book. Even with the help of Jordan's primary doctor and his records, some things still remain cloudy to this day. Thus, while I have done my best in this regard, I must beg forgiveness if there are some mistakes as to when things occurred, what treatments and medications were used and why, and so on. If indeed there are mistakes in the text, they are my own and not anyone else's, and rest assured that they do not affect the overall message of the book, nor the effectiveness of the healing system outlined.

Most important, I will explain how many of these healing principles and methods were applied in Jordan's case and what the startling results were. Do you remember that story about the guy who survived a terminal diagnosis, the one you probably heard when you were little more than a kid yourself? Well, Jordan is *that guy* — the guy who survived. Helping him fight and heal was an experience that changed my life forever, as it did everyone who was close to him. It did so, in part, by teaching us one of life's most powerful lessons, which is that with love all things can be healed.

This lesson is where every true story of healing begins, and so it is where our journey together shall begin as well. It is a journey of self-discovery as much as one of healing, with many lessons to be learned along the way. The fact that love is capable of healing us, mind, body, and spirit, is the first lesson that needs mastering. It is a teaching that came to me during the worst of Jordan's disease, when no hope seemed possible. The words themselves are nothing, and at the time they seemed impossible, too feeble to be trusted — *nice sounding*, but lacking any real power to help. Now I realize how wrong I was. The words were true, then and now, and I have come to believe that they were meant as a gift, not just for Jordan, but for all of us:

With love, all things can be healed; with love, hope is always justified; with love, nothing is impossible — no matter what the doctors tell you.

PART ONE

Principles of Healing

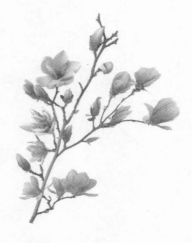

Natural forces within us are the true healers of disease.

— HIPPOCRATES, the father of modern medicine

CHAPTER ONE

Minding Your Mind

*B*efore you can understand all that occurred with Jordan and how his healing came about, it is essential to comprehend some basic principles of the mind-body connection. Often, when a person becomes ill, it requires only a little consideration to uncover the major contributing *nonphysical* elements. When diseases occur, they almost always mirror corresponding dysfunctions on other levels of the patient's life — mental, emotional, spiritual, legal, economic, social, and so on. Furthermore, the larger the physical distress, the more massive the other problems tend to be. In Jordan's case, while he appeared exceptionally healthy in a physical sense before getting sick, there were obvious nonphysical parallels to his disease that were present before the lymphoma itself. The most prominent of these involved his troubled relationship with his divorced parents, who were still living in the same house together, along with Jordan and his older brother.

The specifics of their familial problems do not really matter, and I have chosen not to discuss them in too much detail while telling Jordan's story. The reason for this decision is twofold: First, Jordan has chosen to share a deeply personal story with the world, which is not an easy thing to do. Therefore, when I was able to protect his privacy without omitting key elements of the story or hampering the reader's understanding of the healing process, I have chosen to do so.

Second, as I suggested above, I consider the nature of the conflicts between Jordan and his family to be irrelevant. We all experience conflict, which certainly *does* influence the state of our physical health; however, the particulars aren't important in the least. Jordan's strained relationships were probably not much different than anyone else's. The point is, this book is not a "he said, she said" chronicle that seeks to point fingers or lay blame over causes. Rather, it is a true story about a life-or-death struggle that really occurred and ended happily. The book's main focus is on the key ingredients that allowed healing to happen.

As we will explore, outer conflict is really only a symptom of inner conflict, just as physical distress is a symptom of emotional distress. The forms in which interpersonal conflicts are housed are never the real problem. This is something everyone needs to understand when it comes to relationships. Like the symptoms of any disease, the "issues" that exist between people, and which seem to be the cause of their discord, are actually only *effects* of deeper dysfunctions. This is always true, no matter what type of problem is visible on the surface of the relationship, and it brings up an essential rule of healing that is important enough to qualify as our first major principle.

Principle of Healing I

All diseases — no matter their form — must be treated at the deepest level in order for the condition to be healed.

This principle may sound obvious, but you might be surprised how often it is ignored. All it means is that you cannot cure an illness by treating its symptoms alone. If you had cancer, for instance, you could not heal it merely by taking pills in order to control the pain without actually treating the underlying disease itself — the *cancer*. It can be said that a disease "treated" in this manner is not truly being treated at all. Some illnesses may appear to resolve themselves when dealt with in this way, but all that has really happened is that certain specific symptoms have retreated. Unless the cause of a disease is addressed, it is bound to recur or shift in form. In some cases it may even arise again as a completely different sickness altogether, apparently unrelated to the original distress, but with the same psychical basis.

An additional point is that when we speak of *illness*, we are referring to disease on *all levels*. Suffering comes in many forms. Sickness on the physical plane is only the grossest and most obvious. Disease can also invade an individual's life in just about any area. Dysfunctions of various sorts can disrupt your relationships, work and career, financial and legal situations, sexuality, and so on. Obviously there are also mental and behavioral diseases, which, like physical ones, come in many forms and levels of severity. A few of these are depression, anxiety, obsessive-compulsive behaviors, addictions, eating disorders, panic attacks, rage, narcissism, and psychosis, but there are many other forms of mental illness, and countless variations of each.

On a side note, society has a tendency to take "diseases of the mind" less seriously than physical illnesses, but mental illness can be equally disturbing to a patient's well-being, and sometimes also terminal. On January 21, 2011, a dear friend of mine, the poet Eugene Perri, ended his lifelong struggle with depression by hanging himself to death in his garage while his wife — who is also a close friend — was away at work. While I can still sense Eugene's presence within me, his earthly voice has surely been missed. If nothing else, this type of loss can serve to remind us that mental illness can have many serious, even devastating, consequences, and in order to be truly healthy we must tend to each other's well-being, along with our own, on *every level*, not just the physical.

The universe we live in is not one-dimensional, and neither are you. Therefore, disease in any form, on any level of your being, whether you judge it to be something relatively minor, severe, or even "impossible to heal," should be addressed with equal healing determination. True happiness and health, which actually go hand-in-hand and can never be fully experienced apart, is a *total* experience. Either the state of well-being is present or it is absent, for reason would suggest that "partial health" must imply the presence of "partial disease," which cannot be regarded as total health. Another way of saying this is, *suffering is suffering, whatever the form, level, and cause.*

Yet reason also bids us to ask ourselves what the point is of trading one symptom for another. All that happens when you follow the path of treating an illness from the wrong end — such as through physical treatments of the body exclusively — is to establish a confounding pattern of ever-shifting symptoms, which may occur in a blindingly complex web. It does not matter if you fix one problem; there will always be another right behind it. If not immediately, the wait is unlikely to be long. Each disease does *seem* to have its own unique cause and consequences. How else could the illness remain unhealed when its symptoms have retreated? Left untreated at its root, it *must* change in form or arise again at a later time. In this way a physical illness may shift its outward face many times over many years — in some cases across decades — and it can even transform into a mental disease, or vice versa, and back again. What is the point of chasing shadows?

This is why it is of critical importance to treat the whole person and not just their physical and circumstantial symptoms, including familial dysfunction. Look deeper, into the head and heart of the individual. Symptoms may appear on many levels, but the cause of every illness lies deep within the patient. In Jordan's case, one of his main sources of love had been disrupted due to his difficult relationship with his parents. In particular, as Brittany and Jordan became closer, his connection with his mother grew increasingly rocky, until it reached a state of disarray that mirrored the disaster befalling his body. This eventually became an acute downward cycle: the more troubled his relationship with his mom became, the sicker Jordan got.

Principle of Healing 2
Every thought has an effect on the body.

Another important premise of spiritual therapy that must be clearly understood is that the mind and body are directly connected and influence each other to such a degree that, for practical purposes, they may be considered a solitary, unified system. This is not a conceptual play on words, but a fact. Your feelings and general mood affect your body directly. This influence is easily detectable through various basic measurements. For instance, when you are actively upset, your pulse rate, blood pressure, and respiration may all noticeably increase. These are just a few of the acute physiological changes we can detect using simple medical tools, but there are others. Many of these effects may be subtle, even undetectable day to day, but their impact over time is enormous. For example, if you are chronically stressed, you may gradually develop hypertension, which over decades can lead to heart disease — the number one cause of death in the United States and many other nations.

Likewise, what you experience on a physical level in turn affects your mood, creating a closed system that continuously reinforces itself.

Regardless of your personal spiritual beliefs, when it comes to health and healing, it is helpful to think of your body as a denser, material extension of your mind. As will be explored later, all bodily states have a correlating mental reflection. This doesn't mean that, if you are afraid of developing cancer, you will actually do so. The results of fear thoughts are not generally so specific. What it *does* mean is that there is a strong tendency for negative thought patterns to produce negative consequences in the body. Thoughts are just like everything else in the universe of time and space. That is, they are composed of energy, and energy has a great capacity for creating effects.

Despite the human penchant for viewing diseases as strictly physical phenomena, illnesses actually begin with internal judgments, which cause ripples of negatively charged emotions to spread across the fabric of the mind and out into the body. Essentially this is the same thing that occurs when you drop a stone into a pond and cause little waves to arc out from the point of splashdown. In the mind, these waves are actually comprised of creative energy, and they may be either healing or harming, depending on their nature. Your thoughts, attitudes, beliefs, emotions, judgments, and desires all fuse together with your will to cause a continuous energetic stream of creative potential, which passes through your body and into the world at large.

Much of this theory may at first appear to be just unproven metaphysical conjecture, but it isn't only spiritualists who have observed the connection between the mind and body. Scientists have also documented it. In her book *Molecules of Emotion: The Science Behind Mind-Body Medicine,* Dr. Candace Pert — a pharmacologist with more than 250 published scientific articles and the co-discoverer of the endorphin system — summarized her own research on the subject in the following way: "Mind doesn't dominate body, it becomes body — body and mind are one. I see the process of communication we have demonstrated, the flow of information throughout the whole organism, as evidence that the body is the actual outward manifestation, in physical space, of the mind."

Even if you do not choose to believe that the body and mind are literally one, the influence of thoughts and attitudes on the physical state is hard to deny. A good example of this connection is the fight-or-flight response, which was first identified by Harvard physiologist Walter Bradford Cannon. In simple terms, the fight-or-flight response is a physiological reaction to a perceived threat, whether the threat is real or merely imagined. For instance, when a cat feels threatened by a dog, its hair may stand up on end, its pupils may dilate, and the animal's heart may begin racing, preparing it to either fight the dog or attempt a hasty escape. Of course, this is a natural enough reaction. The cat may very well have to fight for its life, or the dog may mean it no harm. In that moment, however, when confronted with an uncertain situation, the cat's primal instincts kick in and it's not going to take any chances.

It is a *perceived* threat that triggers the response, not necessarily a real threat.

Human beings experience a similar acute response to threatening situations: adrenaline fires into the bloodstream, digestion slows or may even stop, heart rate and respiration soars, certain blood vessels in the body constrict, and vision narrows to the immediate situation. All else vanishes. The reaction is as practical as it is instantaneous and absolute. Imagine crossing a street and seeing a bus racing around the corner: in that moment, you would probably move rapidly, in whatever way was necessary, to save yourself. You wouldn't even need to think about it. The effect can be tremendous. People have been known to leap out of harm's way with inexplicable agility, lift cars weighing thousands of pounds off pinned victims at accident scenes, and fend off bear attacks — all thanks to the fight-or-flight response. In basic physical terms at least, it is a valuable system for helping people survive real, life-threatening emergencies, but problems emerge when it is regularly activated due to trivial, or even imagined, events that don't pose any true threat.

Which brings up an interesting point: the human mind is not particularly good at distinguishing imagined threats from real ones. Perhaps you've noticed that just the thought of conflict can cause your heart rate to increase, your muscles to tighten, and your breath to become shallow and rapid. Indeed, the fight-or-flight response can be activated by the force of your imagination alone and even by minor day-to-day stressors. The reflex itself is neutral. It is intended for emergencies, not in order to compensate for harmful, long-term thinking patterns.

When you honestly examine the relationship between your thoughts and your body, it is easy to see the connection. The bond between the mind and body is so intimate and interwoven, where one begins and the other ends is impossible to distinguish even through serious scientific scrutiny. In simplest terms, this is why filling your mind with stress-causing thoughts makes you more susceptible to physical pathologies. Such thoughts may appear in many forms, such as anger, hatred, jealousy, fear, regret, guilt, greed, envy, sacrifice, victimization, sadness, self-loathing, competition, ego, and many others. The takeaway of all this is simply that consistently harboring negative thoughts causes a lot of stress and tension in the short term, and it can cause sickness of the body over a lifetime.

One more important point to consider is that every thought that crosses your mind has some energetic charge to it, which is either positive or negative. There is no in-between. Thoughts are energy, and energy causes effects. When it comes to the body, *every thought* reinforces either sickness or health. If a thought is positive in nature, it will strengthen the body and cultivate a general state of wellness, or at minimum it will do no harm. If it is negative, it will feed disease. Therefore, if you want to heal your body, you must first heal your mind.

The Waterfall of Thought

Some spiritual teachers recommend that we should dismiss our thoughts as unimportant, and in one sense, this is correct. The shift into the present moment, the origin of healing, does not actually involve thought, or time, or any notion of self-awareness at all. This switch can be performed in any given moment because it is an internal transition into a state of being that is always present, no matter what circumstance you happen to find yourself dealing with. By definition, the present moment cannot be experienced in the future. As long as you believe it can, you will be unable to experience the endless, joyous release that accompanies the state of being. Any given student could achieve so-called enlightenment, which is a state of perfect healing, in any given instant. Even relatively new students along a conscious spiritual path could do so simply by realizing that it is only a single shift in awareness — from a focus on the past and future to an acceptance of the present — that separates them from their goal. The journey to Self realization is indeed short, and being a shift into timelessness, it requires no time at all to accomplish. Any instant will suffice as long as the student is willing.

With this in mind, however, I would like to ask you to try an experiment. Set this book aside and sit quietly for the next few minutes, observing your thoughts. Let your mind wander in whatever direction it feels naturally drawn, but pay attention to the basic content and types of thoughts that cross your mind. Try it now.

The first thing you may notice when you try this exercise is the sheer volume of your thoughts. The average person thinks tens of thousands of thoughts each day. These thoughts begin flowing first thing in the morning, just after you wake up, appearing as a kaleidoscope of words, images, and mingling emotions, which represent your interpretation of everything you see, hear, think, feel, and experience. For most people, the inner dialogue is a virtually unbroken background drone of white noise. This endless stream of thought is what some Buddhists call *the waterfall of thought,* since its presence is as steady as the roar of water cascading over a waterfall.

There are two consequences when this mammoth stream of thought is significantly composed of negative dialogue. First, it induces a fear-laden state, which makes the shift into the present moment, and by extension healing, seem fearful. Fear states actively create mental-emotional blocks to engaging with the present. Second, if your inner dialogue includes many fear-, guilt-, or anger-based thoughts, the body's fight-or-flight response may become chronically activated. Consider that the average person processes roughly sixty thousand thoughts per day. If even 5 percent of these are upsetting or otherwise negative in nature — or what we will collectively refer to as *fear thoughts* from here on out — this means you would be entertaining some three thousand illness-inducing thoughts each day. Multiple this number by 365 and you get your annual dose of fear, which comes out to roughly one million stress-activating, heart-palpitating thoughts per year, every year.

Furthermore, consider that this is a profoundly conservative estimate. Some researchers have suggested that negative thoughts, in one form or another, constitute as much as 50 percent of the average person's thinking process. And we wonder why we get sick.

In human terms, our thoughts are important indeed, and their impact cannot, and should not, be underestimated. The way to repair a waterfall of thought that is mired in negativity does not involve devaluing or dismissing the importance of your thoughts; it involves systematically reprogramming the waterfall itself. Such mind training takes focus, commitment, and great effort to accomplish in full, but fortunately mastery is not necessary in order to receive the benefits of the reprogramming process.

The procedure for retraining your thoughts will be discussed in more detail in chapter 9. For now, you can begin the process by simply becoming aware of your thoughts. Practice taking time every day to observe your mind at random moments, noting the dominant thoughts, emotions, and general patterns that are present, as you did in the above exercise. By bringing consciousness to the waterfall, you begin to identify the areas of your life that cause you the most pain and conflict, and awareness of what needs healing is an essential prerequisite to recovery.

Keep in mind, though, that the thoughts you initially become aware of through this practice by no means represent the full extent of the fear thoughts that inhabit your thinking, many of which may be buried deep in your unconscious mind, but they do provide an obvious place to begin the procedure of rooting them out. Once you understand the impact your thoughts have on your body and emotional state, and you begin to distinguish the difference between thoughts that cause harm from those that support your well-being, your path into conscious healing has begun. This is the first step.

CHAPTER TWO

The Seeds of Disease

*B*efore his bout with lymphoma, Jordan Young was a wiry, seventeen-year-old kid with straight blond hair and an enormous grin, which he was quick to share with the world. After his treatments, his hair became curly and brown, although with every new haircut it is gradually getting closer to its original color. This change occurred as the result of a bone-marrow transplant that Jordan received during the course of his therapy. His blood type also switched due to this brutal and harrowing procedure, flipping virtually overnight to respectively match his donor's characteristics.

Before the lymphoma, Jordan was also a talented snowboarder who could be seen every winter, snow or shine, pulling tricks on the slopes of Mt. Bachelor, near Bend, Oregon. Remarkably, he qualified to compete in the USASA National Championships only months after receiving the above-mentioned transplant. Sadly, due to damage that occurred to his knees during his medical treatments, his ability to snowboard at competitive levels ended not long after this achievement. Although modern medicine has advanced greatly over the past century, negative side effects such as this serve to remind us that we still have a great deal to learn.

More than anything, though, what wins people's hearts is Jordan's playful, easy-going personality, as well as his underlying, boyish innocence. It was one of the first things I sensed about him, and the kid within Jordan still lives, true and strong, despite the trials he's been through. Too often, tragedies of this magnitude stomp the inner life out of a person as disease infiltrates the body, thus damaging a person's body and spirit both. Whoever you are, and whatever your own struggles may be, either now or in the future, whether physical or emotional, above all else you must strive not to allow this ultimate tragedy to occur, for there is no greater loss — including, in my opinion, the death of the body itself. The death of a person's spirit is far greater.

None of this praise is meant to imply that on a behavioral level Jordan was, or is, perfect. He's a bright kid, and like many intelligent youths, he has a mind of his own and the determination to do things his own way. One choice he made on his own was to switch high schools to what is considered an "alternative" public school, Marshall High. His grades were good, and there was no reason for the transfer other than his desire to spend more time on the mountain and less time in the classroom. The liberal setting of Marshall allowed him to take some of his classes online, which freed up his afternoons to hone his snowboarding skills. This choice wouldn't work for every student, but in the end Marshall, with its many devoted teachers and small class sizes, turned out to be an especially good fit. Jordan thrived there, making good grades and close friends with his peers and the school's staff. Marshall is also where he met Brittany and in turn became a part of our family.

Then, in January 2012, when Jordan was a senior, his symptoms first started. A lump the size of a golf ball appeared along

Jordan's neckline, just below his jaw, and he reported feeling physically exhausted and suffering from night sweats that soaked his sheets through.

One of the things his doctor initially tested him for was Hodgkin's disease, a form of lymphoma that occurs most commonly in children and adolescents. That test, however, came back negative, as did several others for prime suspects, including one for pneumonia. Eventually, after more than a month of wasted time, effort, and frustration, the cause behind his distress was discovered: the golf ball turned out to be a swollen lymph node, clogged with cancer cells. Jordan had something called anaplastic large cell lymphoma (ALCL), an aggressive non-Hodgkin's form of the disease, which is relatively rare in people his age. The news was devastating.

Lymphoma is a cancer of the blood, specifically affecting the white blood cells, which are a vital part of the immune system. These precious cells can be thought of as the police officers of the body. Their primary function is to protect us from infections, foreign invaders of various forms, and certain diseases that can arise from within the body itself, such as cancer. White blood cells are born in the bone marrow, which is a flexible tissue at the core of bones, but they exist in every part of the body.

In the case of lymphoma, the white blood cells become cancerous and begin multiplying out of control, subsequently clogging the body's lymph nodes, which function as filters for the lymph system. If left untreated, lymphoma eventually spreads cancerous cells to the body's organs and other tissues — a process that may be either very slow or blindingly rapid, depending on the type of lymphoma and the particular case. This interrupts the normal workings of the body and starves its tissues and organs of nutrients and oxygen, thus destroying them and eventually killing the patient.

Jordan had been diagnosed at Stage 3 of the disease process, which indicated that the cancer had already grown and started to spread significantly. Stage 4, the most serious stage, occurs when the illness begins invading organs and tissues far beyond those it originated in. Eventually this spread becomes out of control and irreversible. Little did we realize when Jordan was first diagnosed that it would be only a few tumultuous months before he would become deeply entrenched in Stage 4, and not long after that considered most likely terminal.

Dr. Bill Martin is an oncologist at St. Charles Cancer Center in Bend, Oregon, and after Jordan's diagnosis, he became the primary doctor in charge of Jordan's care. Dr. Martin started Jordan right away on a standard chemotherapy drug known as CHOP, which was administered via injection. At the outset, Dr. Martin expressed optimism regarding Jordan's chances for surviving the disease. Jordan was young, and youth is a major asset when it comes to healing, especially in the case of lymphomas. When Jordan began treatment, everyone who was close to him was hopeful. We all assumed he would get through this trial, frightening as it was, with relative ease.

Chemo drugs are toxic stuff, literally. Actually, their toxicity is how they destroy cancer. These "medications" are designed to attack the body's cells, in particular those that divide rapidly, which is a part of cancer's primary dysfunction — wild, out-of-control mitosis. This is what makes chemo especially effective at killing cancer cells. The problem is that chemo also indiscriminately destroys *healthy* fast-multiplying cells. In the human body, these types of cells are primarily located in the digestive system, bone marrow, and hair, which is why chemo patients may become prone to other, secondary infections during treatment, since the body's primary defenders — fast-multiplying white blood cells — are destroyed in large numbers by the drugs. It also accounts for the reason patients often lose their hair. Chemotherapy has made baldness one of the tell-tale signs of cancer. Some people think the disease causes the hair loss, but it's the drugs. The objective when treating cancer with chemotherapy, of course, is to kill the mutant cancerous cells without killing the patient. Suffice it to say, this process presents a decidedly tricky balancing act.

For some cancer patients, losing their hair is embarrassing, but as with all things in life, patients are wise to learn the art of reinterpreting apparent negative effects in a positive light. This is true no matter what the sickness, symptoms, side effects, and treatments happen to be. In the case of losing one's hair, for instance, a patient might choose to view this change as a symbol of courage, strength, and determination to heal. In this way it becomes a sort of badge of honor, as opposed to a symbol of weakness and disease.

This is not to suggest that watching such physical changes take place is easy. As Jordan began his treatment, his youthful, shaggy mane thinned and gradually dropped from his head, and something in the sudden shift seemed to cause his sickness to harden and become more real to both him and everyone else. It is difficult to accept a diagnosis as scary as his. It's like getting sucker punched. You're just not ready for it. Nobody ever is. Diseases like this invariably seem to strike from nowhere, although this is anything but true. The psychical roots of disease are in place well before the disease manifests in the body. The physical appearance of an illness is, nevertheless, typically stunning. At first you may feel shocked into a sort of numbness, unable to process what is happening. Then, as the numbness wears off, the retreat into fear begins. Of course, you want to stay optimistic, and you are told by virtually everyone that you *must*, but for almost every patient and their loved ones, fear becomes the very first obstacle that needs to be surmounted.

Coping with Fear

For those readers who have come to this book due to illness, I would like to ask you to pause right now, close your eyes for a moment, and make the following commitment to yourself. Say:

I will get through this. I will be well. I will recover.

Repeat this statement several times, slowly, with as much focus as possible. Try to feel the words settling within you, hardening, and becoming real. Above all else, do your best to believe them — no matter what you are facing and what you have been told.

For those readers with a loved one who is ill, take his or her hands in your own, set aside any fear you may have, and as sincerely as possible, tell her or him the following:

I am with you. You are not alone. We will get through this — together. You will recover.

Whether patient or supporter, resolve yourself to this declaration. Attempt to sense the strength behind the words you are speaking or thinking, and keep them firmly in mind as your journey proceeds. Remind yourself of them daily. You cannot wish disease away, hide from it, or deny its presence in your life, just as you cannot deny negative thinking habits. You must first acknowledge your present situation, but at the same time recognize that through your acceptance your journey becomes one of conscious healing, not deepening sickness, even if your path *appears* to lead you in the other direction at the outset. All healing begins with the determination to heal. What this means is, if you want to achieve any goal, the first step is to *desire* its achievement. Just as cancer progresses through various stages, so too does the healing process, and the decision to get better could rightly be labeled *Stage 1* of healing. It is a decision that is most powerful when made consciously, with real desire and conviction fueling it.

Realize, too, that the only way to successfully traverse the path before you without fear is by taking one deliberate step at a time, while remaining focused on *just that step*. This is the key to dealing with fear. It is essential to train yourself not to project into the future. Dedicate yourself, fully and without reserve, to allowing each day to be the most important, precious thing to you, while you are experiencing it. Don't focus on what hasn't arrived, nor on what has passed. Forget about the future and the past both. If you wish to be at peace and find hope, joy, and meaning during the healing process, you cannot live for tomorrow nor for the days that have gone by. On the road to recovery, you must learn to leave tomorrow's worries for tomorrow, or you will *never* be free of fear, and your healing — or your loved one's healing — will be hampered as a result. Difficult as this objective may appear, there is no way around it, and yet you may find that it is not as hard as it at first sounds. Once you begin challenging yourself to stay grounded in the here and now, you will discover a light-heartedness and an easy joy that will reinforce your every effort.

What you must understand and accept unreservedly is that fear is a direct antagonist to healing, therefore it needs to be dealt with directly, not hidden away, covered over with denial, or forced into unconsciousness. It comes from worrying about a future that you can neither predict nor control.

Leave the future to God, and let your only concern be today, right now, this very moment. In the space of the present lies your total, and immediate, release from the bondage of fear.

Principle of Healing 3
Fear thoughts feed disease.

This principle expands on the last one, taking it one step further, and it is a central, connecting idea that links all the remaining principles together. If there is one thing that can be said of every one of our healing principles, thus unifying them, it is that they are all based on the premise that *healing begins within, in the head and heart of the patient.* Indeed, this thought adequately summarizes the entire driving philosophy behind the healing system. It suggests that while there may be physical treatments involved in any given healing, such as medications, surgeries, and the like, it is really what happens in the mind of the patient that determines whether such treatments will be successful in triggering healing.

Various healers over the centuries have noted that *love heals*, but it is equally true that hatred sickens. This is how the seeds of disease can hide inside our own mind without us ever realizing we are actually poisoning ourselves. Most people never even suspect that their thoughts and feelings are the primary cause behind every form of ill they will ever suffer. For hatred is a personal thing, a thought that, once it occurs, is then cherished by the thinker, in the same way a mother is bound to love her own child. It is natural for you to care for your creations, which include your thoughts and beliefs, not just your biological offspring. This effect remains in force even when those creations are inherently unworthy and cause you pain and suffering. For this precise reason people have a strong tendency to covet, and even actively defend, illness-producing thinking.

You may believe that sickness is something that happens only to your body, and that it is caused by mysterious forces that lie outside of you, or perhaps by forces hidden within the body's internal structure and awaiting the right conditions to manifest, but certainly not caused by your own mind. Thus, you may believe illness is beyond your ability to control. I'd encourage you to challenge any beliefs regarding this notion. If you realized the sweeping power of your mind, and the influence your thoughts have over the condition of your body, you would see at once that you could, at a very minimum, assist your body in healing to a degree you have never imagined. The affect of your mind and attitude on the body is precisely what makes laughter such a potent medication, and love, without a doubt, the greatest healer of them all.

Yet your thoughts, moods, and feelings do much more than merely affect your body. As previously alluded to, when disease appears on the physical plane, there is *always* an emotional parallel, or reflection, to the illness in the patient's mental sphere. Furthermore, if the mental-emotional aspect of an illness is cured, the physical part will naturally fix itself — *somehow, someway*. A treatment that had not worked before will suddenly begin working; the right medication will be found; the perfect healer will show up at the perfect moment, drawn into the patient's life by one of those mysterious "co-incidences"; or perhaps the patient will spontaneously heal.

During Jordan's journey there came a moment when all hope seemed absolutely, irrevocably lost; when modern medicine could offer no further answers; when his young journey through life appeared to be a journey into death. Yet precisely at this same moment, when the world's ineffective answers to his disease had clearly failed, one by one, true healing and hope were born anew. It was a terrible moment, to be sure, saturated with fear and darkness and the grim, cold certainty of death. And yet here is where Jordan reached his turning point away from sickness, and grimness, and death, and shifted instead into the light of inner healing.

Everyone must reach this stage, or something resembling it: when there is a distinct shift in attitude away from the acceptance of sickness and death and toward embracing healing and life.

There is a moment in every patient's struggle — a flash of light and healing that streaks across the mind — when the person chooses healing. It is a moment that engages the patient fully, on every level. It happens so fast it may not even be remembered afterward; frequently it is not. Yet after that instant is achieved, whether or not it is held in conscious memory, the means for healing will present itself. This healing moment is the goal of all worthwhile treatments.

Whatever the means of healing turn out to be, the process is initiated by helping the patient heal his or her heart and head, a connected sphere that contains our thoughts, attitudes, emotions, spirit, and all other mental and emotional energies, in order for the patient to reach this healing moment. Through purifying these forces, healing is welcomed instead of resisted, brought forth instead of repelled. In an instant, all the patient's struggles give way and the overwhelming force of healing is held off no longer. Healing is natural. The body wants to heal; only the mind resists. So the patient must be helped to unreservedly choose life. This is all healers ever really do, and all healing really requires.

If today's healthcare system has one major flaw, it is the tendency to overlook the spiritual and mental needs of the patient, often *entirely*, in favor of treating physical symptoms alone. This style of treatment is insufficient no matter what the distress, as it addresses only one dimension of our being — specifically, the body — which itself represents only the grossest, most basic element of what we are. Each human lifetime is a dance between the spiritual, mental, and physical aspects of the individual. Therefore treating any one of these parts while ignoring the others can never completely succeed in healing. Once again, in order to heal you must treat the *whole person*, not just one part.

I'd like to invite you to take this point, put it into your head, and don't ever forget it! This truth is guaranteed to serve you well, and faithfully, in countless situations.

One other thing that needs mentioning here is that this view is not meant to diminish the role that medical professionals play in helping a patient to heal. In this world, more often than not, healing will *seem* to be a complicated, challenging, and time-consuming procedure. All true helpers are needed and welcomed in this process, and each one performs a specific role that he or she is best suited for. In Jordan's case, many of the doctors and nurses who attended him deserve our deepest thanks. Without their help, care, and mastery of the human body, Jordan's journey might have ended just as it was getting started. Yet it cannot be denied that a holistic approach to healing is essential if it is to be complete, and this needs to include a balanced treatment plan involving all appropriate medical, spiritual, and emotional therapies. If a patient does not want to live, what good does healing the body do? The person will just become ill again, at some point down the road. The outcome, selected by the individual's own will, is inevitable.

If you are currently receiving medical or psychiatric care, taking medications, or undergoing any other physical remedies, it is recommended that you continue to do so as long as you and your doctor, or other involved professionals, agree that they are useful. The techniques in this book are not intended to replace such treatments. Indeed, many of us are so used to relying on physical remedies that a truly unexplained — entirely psychical — healing might trigger panic, which is a blatantly counterproductive reaction. It is sometimes gentler to allow medications, healers, and "procedures" as such to adopt healing characteristics. Do not forget that Source, being unlimited, works through everyone and everything in our world in order to help us heal, including our doctors, nurses, psychologists, medications, procedures, and so on. Healing attempts that utilize these things and people are therefore not inherently "anti-spiritual," as some people regard them. They are best thought of as temporary aids to assist the healing process or tools that provide a means to reach the desired goal of recovery.

Resistance to Healing

The fact that many patients are actually afraid of healing does not appear to make much sense when stated directly. After all, who, in the throes of sickness and pain, would fear to be healed? The answer may surprise you as much as it did me: everyone who is suffering, in any way, degree, or form, is afraid of healing. And *yes*, sadly, I do include myself in this list!

You may experience significant resistance to this idea at first. I know I did, and I still do from time to time. I encourage you, however, no matter what your initial reaction may be, to try your best to set aside your own opposition and consider this notion thoroughly.

In this world, to the sick and suffering, nothing is more fearful than healing. Actually, deep mental resistance to healing is the *primary* obstacle the sick and dying face. It is the same type of bizarre, counterproductive reaction that some people have to success. The driving cause behind the fear is that, in the ultimate sense, healing involves spiritual awakening, and virtually all of us have a deep-seated fear of enlightenment, albeit an unconscious one. If you didn't have any fear of awakening, you would instantly awaken. Only fear holds enlightenment off. For this same reason sickness is often used as an unconscious means to reinforce the false disconnect from Spirit that characterizes life on earth. The state of illness accomplishes this by emphasizing our connection to the body through pain and discomfort, thus anesthetizing us to our reality as spiritual beings.

Anyone who has ever had a legitimate spiritual revelation understands that during the mystical experience, the body is risen beyond and temporarily lost touch with. Some people describe this as a sense of "numbness," but the body does not actually become numb during revelation. Rather, your focus shifts away from it and you rise beyond it. In part, physical pain and disease are a way of clinging to our corporeal boundaries out of the fear of what lies beyond the body. This is precisely why advanced spiritual people sometimes become sick, too.

So it is that the healing moment comes like a revelation when, for just one instant, the patient releases fear and forgets the physical self entirely, rising beyond it and into the sphere of Spirit. In this way, the fear and sickness are simultaneously surmounted in precisely the same manner and at precisely the same instant.

This is why it is critical for all patients to remember — and to remind themselves continuously until it becomes a habit of thinking — that there is nothing to be feared in awakening. You cannot be endangered in any manner, or by any means, by reconnecting with your true Self or with Source. You can go as deeply as you like into the Divine space, and you will never be attacked or injured in any way; just the opposite. Even your ego will remain quite intact upon your return to ordinary consciousness. Only your perspective will have shifted, and always for the better.

Finally, the idea that healing begins within a person's heart and head is not intended to place the "blame" for an illness on the patient's shoulders. Blame in general is utterly pointless, and it certainly serves no purpose where healing is concerned. There is no circumstance in which it is helpful, particularly when someone is sick. This stance does not mean that we should ignore obvious self-destructive behavior, but we must strive to recognize that blame is not needed in order to identify and correct errors. As we will explore, blame and guilt — which is blame turned inward and used against oneself — are directly adversarial to the healing process. These emotions, and a few others, are highly destructive to the body, and they contribute greatly to disease by feeding it directly.

The seeds of sickness exist within us all. Everyone in this world has some underlying potential for disease, so no one need feel ashamed or guilty about becoming sick. On the contrary, by acknowledging the role we play in creating our own illness, we are turning in the direction of healing, and we can accept responsibility for our state with relief and a sigh of thanks, for it stands to reason that if we can cause ourselves to become sick, we must also possess the power to heal.

The Garden of the Body

With all this in mind, in order to heal, it is thus vital to learn to identify illness-producing thinking. We have already stated that fear thoughts, in their various forms, are major disease contributors. Now let's consider this relationship more directly and identify what these thoughts look like.

The *content* of fear thoughts can be just about anything. They are usually words or images that focus on something that has occurred in the past or is anticipated in the future; they are any thoughts that center around judgment, grievances, anger, hatred, violence, anxiety, sadness, grief, guilt, racism, shame, weakness, vulnerability, victimization, worry, competitiveness, greed, or the many other masks ego may wear. In short, they are always focused on the bad, never on the good, and they typically increase our sense of differentness and separation from others.

It may be helpful to think of your body as a garden, your mind as the gardener, and your thoughts as the seeds you plant. Each thought that crosses your mind affects your mental state as well as your physical well-being, whether or not you are aware of the thought. Not every negative seed necessarily gives rise to illness, not directly anyway, but when large numbers of them infiltrate any one area, or intense emotional wounds are left to fester instead of being forgiven and healed, disease is bound to occur in one form or another.

Therefore you must become a conscientious gardener of your life, planting only the crops that yield peace, happiness, and health, while weeding out those that cause harm, many of which may already be present in your mind. Ask yourself, in open honesty, what areas in your life cause you the most distress, anger, fear, guilt, and so on. What pushes your buttons? I mean, what — and who — *really* pisses you off? Whatever those areas are, these harbor the greatest propensity for creating illness. The process of cultivating health involves learning how to forgive your ancient hurts and grievances, one by one, which simply means that you find some way — in your own mind — to look upon them with a sense of peace, acceptance, and release, rather than judgment, animosity, and intolerance.

This process does involve some discipline at first, until it becomes a set pattern and way of life. You begin by simply *deciding* to begin. In other words, you set your intention to do so. Next, each day remind yourself that you are now becoming a conscious "gardener." Start today, right now. Pause for a moment and determine to be an intentional architect of your life, which includes the thoughts you allow to remain unchallenged in your mind.

Next, reinforce this intention each day in this same manner. With every new morning remind yourself of the types of seeds you want to plant; the emotions you *want* to experience; the things you would like to think about during the passage of each day, realizing their monumental impact on you. There is no real need to tell yourself what to avoid. Merely focus on the positive, and when something does not fit in, you will easily learn to identify it, just as a real gardener can distinguish a weed from a carrot even at a distance.

You will further need to remind yourself of your new purpose throughout the day, ideally reinforcing it at regular intervals. If it helps, set up a schedule that is easy to remember. For instance, you might make a point of pausing to examine your thoughts and clear out those that don't mesh with your goal whenever you eat, or take a drink of water, or at the top of every passing hour. Or wear a bracelet, a ring, or even just a rubber band that serves to remind you of your intention every time you notice it. The point is to establish some cue that will remind you to periodically stop and clear out negative thoughts at regular intervals.

If you are ever unsure which thoughts contribute to health, and which to disease, simply remember that disease-producing thoughts *always* create a sense of discomfort in one form or another, whether emotional discord or physical distress. Meanwhile, healing thoughts are *always* accompanied by joy and a sense of unity, peace, and cooperation with others. In any instant, you can identify the form of each thought by asking yourself, honestly, "How do I feel right now?" Are you happy? Joyous? Do you feel connected to the people around you, satisfied, safe, and loved? If your answer to any of these questions is *no*, even if your sense of pain is minor, there must be a fear thought lurking in your head and heart that needs to be dealt with.

You will find many of these as you go along. Rooting them

out is the work of healing; indeed, it is the work of life — it is why you are here, enrolled in Earth School.

Principle of Healing 4
Love thoughts heal.

The opposite of fear thoughts are *love thoughts*. These represent all the thoughts that bring a sense of quietness, joy, and acceptance to you. Like fear thoughts, love thoughts come in many forms, but also like fear thoughts, their form is not what matters. They are easy to identify if you pay attention to your feelings, which are the result of your thoughts. Love thoughts may reflect or evoke compassion, understanding, joy, acceptance, forgiveness, gentleness, unity, cooperation, charity, nonjudgment, and gratitude, among other qualities. The importance of love thoughts lies, not so much in their manner of expression, but in the energetic charge they infuse your emotional and physical bodies with. Each one, in its own unique way, invites and reinforces love, which makes you aware of your connection with others and with Source. This is why even the simplest expressions of love are so infused with healing potential, just as fear thoughts are vessels of disease. When you are actively giving and receiving love, it is impossible to be afraid, to feel abandoned, or to hate and attack. With love in your perception, you automatically stop focusing on faults and mistakes — whether yours or another's — and start focusing on the things that are right and good about life. And when problematic behavior *does* need addressing, you are more likely to switch into problem-solving mode rather than engaging in finger-pointing.

Love also opens our eyes to compassion and gratitude. Compassion helps us understand that those who are locked into a pattern of fear and anger are actually in desperate need. They are suffering, and what they truly require is healing, not counterattack and hatred. This can be challenging to remember in the face of attack, but it nevertheless reflects an unalterable law of healing, which states that it is impossible to heal hatred with hatred. This would be like trying to cure cancer with cancer. Does such a mad prescription make any sense when put into simple terms like this? Of course it doesn't. The only way to heal *anything* is with its opposite. So the only way to heal hatred, in whatever form it occurs, is with love. Prejudice requires acceptance; rage may be successfully defeated only by calmness; pettiness is undone by grandeur; bullying gives way when it is met with courage; vindictiveness is healed through compassion; when ingratitude meets a grateful heart, the power of thankfulness stands out so bright, and so clear, that it cannot be denied; and tyrants must be disbanded by the quiet presence of love.

It is notable, too, that disease-causing emotions simply cannot coexist with the state of love because love is absolute. Like fear, its opposite, love is experienced completely in any given instant or it is not felt at all. You may rapidly shift back and forth between these two emotions, but if you monitor your feelings with precision, you will observe that love and fear can never be present together in the same space at the same instant. Because of this, when any thought of fear, guilt, or anger enters your mind, love may seem to disappear, but we say *seem* here only because love has not really departed. What you are in truth is made of love, or at least that is the approximate comparison in worldly terms that virtually every mystic, of every spiritual tradition, throughout recorded history has consistently reported. Words can never describe what you are in truth, but *love* is a close enough comparison. What has actually occurred when love seems to be shut out from your life, and fear rules in its place, is that *you* have turned away from it. Love never dims, shifts, nor wavers, but shines steadily across all of creation, infusing the universe with joy and renewed life with every passing instant. This is not just my personal opinion. You can learn to feel and directly experience this for yourself.

As your awakening deepens, you are bound to shift back and forth between states of loving and fearing, peace and war, forgiveness and contempt. Even great sages experience this confounding, and painful, pattern. You shouldn't feel disappointed or guilty when you find yourself grappling with the urge to hate, attack, and judge. Instead, focus on becoming deeply aware of just one stunning revelation that has the power to transform your life forever: that is, fear thoughts will *always* bring you pain, no matter how justified your anger seems to be. It is *you* who will suffer and experience guilt in response to every attack — no matter how slight — that you make upon another. Also, you must come to a clear and unshakable understanding that love thoughts, in sharp contrast to fear thoughts, always elicit joy. Learn this and you have learned all that you will ever need to know about the journey of awakening.

True Love versus False Love

To clarify, when we speak of love as a healing device, we are not referring to romantic love necessarily. True healing love can exist in any relationship, with any living creature. The specific roles of those involved do not matter. Love is a state of union in which two or more seemingly separate beings choose each other, without judgment, and become aware of their oneness. This experience feels much the same as the healing instant.

The sense of connection may be brief, lasting no more than a moment, a fraction of a fraction of an instant. Often those united in this union do not even realize anything out of the ordinary has occurred. Rest assured, however, that lack of awareness will not hinder the ultimate effect of the experience, although developing the ability to *consciously* experience this union is certainly worthwhile. This deeply healing experience can be greatly amplified if it is kept in awareness and not allowed to be swept into oblivion by the passage of time or covered over by fear thoughts.

Unfortunately, many relationships, romantic or otherwise, are based on resentment and hatred, whether frank or veiled, but clearly not on love and unity. We are not referring to these destructive relationships, which actually *exclude love*. A good rule of thumb is, if a relationship arouses more pain than joy, it is itself in need of healing. *How could it serve to heal when it remains unhealed?* Once again we come to the basic law of healing that sickness cannot heal sickness; only its opposite can provide a lasting remedy.

It might sound like a line to say that *love heals* — "impossible," even — but do not read this lightly. I have come to believe that love is the single most important ingredient in the human arsenal for healing illnesses of every type. No pill can equal the natural healing force contained in love. Purified, unconditional love is the highest emotion human beings are capable of. The closer you come to this state, the deeper your healing will be, as well as your propensity to assist others in healing.

Therefore the first thing to ensure when a person becomes sick is that he or she is giving and receiving love freely. The more the person becomes an open channel for loving thoughts, loving attitudes, and loving actions, the more likely healing will occur. The form of the exchange doesn't matter any more than the particular form of illness does, nor do the roles of those involved in the exchange. Love given and received through a dog, for example, is just as effective a healer as love given and received by people. This is why many healing centers and hospitals now encourage patients to spend time with their pets during treatment.

Once again we see the common theme reflected that form does not matter. It is the content behind the form that counts.

Giving and Receiving Love

One additional note regarding love as a healing device needs addressing. On the surface, the giving of love seems to be something quite different than the receiving of love. But look more carefully at this relationship and you may recognize a curious truth: the act of giving and receiving love are inseparably linked in such a manner that — in any given exchange, no matter how large or small, trivial or important, and regardless of the formal roles and relationships that exist — both participants are equally blessed when love is shared. In this way, for practical purposes at least, giving and receiving love are identical.

This is because it is actually Source energy (the Holy Spirit, or *Chi* — it goes by various names) that heals, and love is the human emotion that resonates most closely with Source. Chi is the creative energy that flows throughout the universe. By its very nature it repairs, blesses, and readjusts *everything* it comes into contact with. Whatever needs fixing, Chi operates as the reparative force of nature. For this reason, as Chi passes through the giver, he or she is being healed by it just as much as the so-called recipient. It does not matter what the nature of the distress is, the complexity of the problem, or who is in need of healing. Source energy makes no distinctions among problems or people, size or complexity. It is thoroughly unbiased. Where Source energy flows, it naturally sets *all things* right, which simply means that it returns them to their natural order.

This concept may be difficult to grasp at first because we are used to the idea that we have less of whatever we give away. Of course, this is true of material possessions. For instance, if you give five dollars to a homeless person, you will have five fewer dollars. However, in this experience, more than money is exchanged. By helping a fellow human being in need, you deepen your sense of compassion, and this adds to the richness of your own life in a way that far exceeds monetary value. Therefore you *have* received something valuable in return, even though it came in a different form.

The message here is that in a universe made of energy, nothing is ever lost. This is not an opinion but a scientific fact. Energy does not dissipate. Sunlight streams into the world and feeds the plants of the earth that, in turn, provide food for the animals of the world, which will one day return to the earth's soils and themselves become fodder for the endless cycle of life. Sunlight also warms the water of the seas, setting them into motion and sending moisture into the air, to be carried along the currents of the wind and deposited along mountainsides, jungles, and across cityscapes. As rivers then form, they carry life-sustaining water and energy to the people, insects, animals, plants, and trees that inhabit our world. We don't ordinarily see this cycle happening, but it goes on continuously. Life may shift and change, grow and shrink; it may flourish and, apparently, even perish, but in reality it is but the dance of forms that fools our eyes. Nothing is ever truly lost in this kaleidoscopic, Cosmic play.

CHAPTER THREE

Mind Over Matter

*I*n this world, some things appear possible and other things not. We learn this from a very young age. Gravity, arguably, presents us with our first obvious piece of evidence. *Birds can fly; human beings cannot.* I learned this lesson from an aspen tree that towered above my two-story, childhood home. I was probably only five or six years old the first time I fell from one of its branches and was soundly slammed back to earth, compliments of gravity.

The lesson was instantly acquired. *People can't fly! Okay, I get it.* At least not without assistance. Yet today, people *do* fly every day, all over the world — by plane, helicopter, and other less-traditional means. So in a sense, we *have* overcome gravity. In fact, we did so in a most spectacular display when Commander Neil Armstrong and his crew blasted free of Earth's atmosphere during 1969's Apollo 11 mission to the moon.

What is possible and what is not? Do you think you know? There are many facts that might challenge your preconceived notions. It might sound impossible, for instance, to hold your breath while underwater for much longer than a minute, and for most people it would be impossible. But how much of this effect is due to our beliefs? As of this writing, the world record for such a feat is held by a German free diver who remained underwater for twenty-two minutes.

On a completely different track, when Paramahansa Yogananda — a great meditation teacher and author of the spiritual classic *Autobiography of a Yogi* — died in 1952, his body was said to have remained in a "state of immutability" for weeks, during which it "exhibited no sign of decay," according to the director of Forest Lawn Mortuaries, which handled his body. This is a well-documented case, and there hasn't been any widely accepted rational explanation for it. Other saint's bodies have displayed the same phenomenon, an effect that has been dubbed "the incorruptible body."

There are many things that seem impossible, or which we do not understand, that turn out to be quite feasible after all. Here is one more example, which brings up an intriguing notion: before the year 1954, it was considered "impossible" to run a mile in under four minutes, which gave rise to the notion of a four-minute barrier. In the spring of 1954, however, a British runner named Roger Bannister broke the four-minute barrier when he ran a mile in three minutes and fifty-nine seconds. The really interesting part of this story is that only a few weeks later another runner from Australia also achieved the same goal, besting Bannister's time by less than one second. By this point in history, runners around the globe had been attempting to break the four-minute mile for decades to no avail. These days it is a common enough accomplishment. So it appears as if once the *mental barrier* to the four-minute mile had been conquered, the physical part happened naturally for many athletes.

The point is that when it comes to limits it is difficult to distinguish genuine physical realities — such as, *people can't fly because people don't have wings* — from those constructed by the mind. Of course, really tenacious people don't allow even true physical limitations to deter them. Orville and Wilbur Wright, for instance, did not let the silly fact that they had no wings stop them from taking to the air. They built their own damn wings.

Once more I ask, what is possible and what is not? Do you think you know? In truth, you probably *do know,* but what you may not realize is that you have set up your own limitations. If you believe in them, they will seem to be true — *for you.* But if you refuse to believe in them, you will free yourself to go beyond them, into the open realm of possibility.

The lesson here is simple: be careful about what you believe, for the mind, as has been emphasized, is extraordinarily powerful. Do not accept limitations, no matter who is feeding them to you and how knowledgeable that person may appear. This holds true for the journey of healing, too. To help you rise beyond every self-imposed restriction you may have set up in your mind — anything that may appear to hold you back in any capacity — I invite you to remind yourself of the following thought again and again until it becomes a background mantra in your mind:

There are no limits; it is never too late.

Principle of Healing 5
You are a natural-born creator.

In order to understand just how what is happening inside your head and heart can hurt or heal your body, you must appreciate how powerful you are. You are a creator by nature. In effect, you are *always* creating. Every instant, every day, whether you are awake or asleep, you are actively shaping and reacting to the events of your life. Creating is not a matter of choice, and it has nothing to do with "free will." Free will means only that you get to choose *what* you create, not whether to create or not create. Nor can you change the essence of what you are.

Your soul was born through an act of creation, and that is why you truly are a "natural-born creator," in a literal sense. This is the same as saying you must be like that which gave birth to you. If you owned a pregnant dog, you wouldn't expect it to give birth to a litter of kittens, would you? This is only obvious. But what many do not realize is that it represents a principal tenet of the act of creation, which is that life can only give birth to that which is like itself, or in its own image. In a simple sense this is also ultimately why negative thoughts create negative physical consequences, just as positive ones create in their likeness as well.

Your "true Self," with a capital *S*, is composed of the essence of *That* which gave birth to it — or *Source* — and likewise your own creations also resemble you. Not physically, perhaps, but at the core of their existence. All beings have a core Self, which represents the essence of one's life, and which exists unbound and independently of the ego and physical body both. Your core Self is the original spark from which all else in your life grows. It is like the seed that buds and develops into a plant, which then sprouts with leaves and blossoms with flowers. Your Self is made of the pure creative Chi of the universe, raw and undefined, like a sculptor's clay.

Chi, then, is what you are — your essence — and your body is nothing more than an extension of it, a creative stroke of your will.

Although Chi is the part of you that supplies the energy behind all of your own creations, it is only the raw fuel. You must decide *how* to put it to use, just as an artist must choose canvas, brush, and colors with care. Your creations in time and space are literally extensions of what you believe you are — your deepest held mental abstracts of yourself and your life, which may be, and generally *are*, gravely warped. It is a certainty that what people believe to be true versus what is *actually* true are often out of alignment. Whether factual or not, beliefs are powerful creative forces that are always at work in your life, whether or not you are aware of it. Even now you are using the force of your Chi to manifest your life as it is unfolding in the present moment, here on earth, whenever and wherever you happen to be reading this.

In most people, this process of creation occurs unconsciously. That is why people believe their lives are dependent on the winds of fate, the laws of medicine, and the grace of genetic design. They create, but they do not realize they are creating. Thus the sick do not perceive the role they play in contributing to their disease, nor can they choose healing until their role as pilot of their destiny is recognized and accepted.

Learning to create consciously, then, is a major step toward seizing control of your life and shaping your experience in Earth School as you would prefer it to be. You are not weak and incapable nor the victim of the whims of worldly forces, whether those forces are of human design or natural origins. You are a cocreator of all you see, touch, think, feel, and experience. Your mind and your will are the most powerful forces in the universe — too powerful to allow them to be directed by unconscious motives, whims, and guilt-driven emotions. Your will is powerful enough to summon catastrophe into your life or to shower you with blessings that have no boundaries and no end. It is no idle force. Therefore you must learn to wield it both consciously and wisely.

Principle of Healing 6

**Healing cannot be forced on the patient.
It must be actively invited and openly received.**

Nobody really wants to be sick. Inevitably, those who become ill will pray — on some level, in whatever manner suits them according to their belief system — to get better. This does not imply that the prayer must be set in a religious context. Even a "wish" to heal is a form of prayer. Also, at one time or another, everyone who falls ill and thus prays for healing experiences disappointment should they fail to recover. This is often viewed as evidence that prayer does not work, that there is no God, or that — if there is — God either does not care about human suffering or, even worse, is using disease to punish "sinners."

Two points must be understood, and understood clearly, regarding this particularly murky topic. One: *The roots of disease are often — indeed, virtually always — hidden in unconsciousness.* Just as a plant's roots are usually hidden beneath the ground, so too the roots of disease. It is rarely, if ever, apparent to the patient just how and why they have contributed to their own disease, but when suffering is present, reason would dictate that its roots must be present as well, even if they are hidden from view. It must be so. A tree does not grow with no roots to secure it and take up the nutrients it needs in order to live. For healing to be successful, whether through prayer, medicine, or some other means, above all else the patient must seek to uncover those roots.

Two: *Healing cannot be forced.* It is not that God is cruel, intentionally ignoring some cries for help while answering others, or trying to punish anyone (even those who, in worldly terms, appear to deserve punishment). All those who have had a direct encounter with the presence of God realize that the Great Spirit is incapable of attack on any level, in any way, being composed of perfect, Divine Love. Attack, hatred, and punishment are characteristics of the ego, not of God. When you encounter God, you find yourself so filled with a sense of light, unconditional love, and deepest care, you never want the experience to end. It is unlike any worldly sensation you have ever felt. Yet if an individual is inwardly resistant to healing on *any level*, whether or not the person is conscious of that resistance, Spirit cannot force help that has not been openly invited, no matter how much love God has for us. Doing so would essentially be a form of attack. This, in simple terms, is why sometimes healing is not achieved.

All worldly healers must learn to approach healing with the same care and understanding that God does. If you are supporting someone who is ill, this means that you should not attempt to impose yourself or force your "love" on the patient in any way. Doing so is not *love*. It is a form of attack, and it is impossible that love could be received through force of any kind. Love and attack are opposites in every way and can never be found together. Bullying, coercion, and the many types of manipulation by which egos wage war upon one another, oftentimes in the name of "love" or justified as "best for the patient," are too numerous to even attempt to list here. The world is filled with examples. The one thing they all have in common is that not a single one shares any of the gentle characteristics that attend love.

If a person is actively resistant to receiving love and the healing it brings, the quiet presence of a healer can still be of help. Giving love does not necessarily have anything to do with your actions or words. Authentic love — and in truth there is no other kind — represents a completely nonjudgmental, unconditional connection with another living being. It is a *direct experience*. This can be expressed silently just as readily as through actions and words. I believe that much of the healing that occurred during Jordan's illness was brought about through holding silent presence at his bedside. Loving actions and words themselves merely reflect an internal state of loving *intent*.

Whatever the concern, and wherever healing is needed, do not let any confusion distract you from the difference between love and force, and above all remember this: The words you speak do not matter. Your actions do not matter. You must become an open channel for love and allow it safe and free passage through you and into the heart and head of the one in need. That is all. If you attempt to add more, you will take away from the true Cause of all healing, which is God, not you. This thought brings us to our final Principle of Healing...

Principle of Healing 7

Total healing can occur only through entering the healing dimension, which is a state of direct union with Source.

This final principle ties together everything we have so far discussed. It is curious how much faith human beings place in medicine as opposed to Source energy. This is a particularly odd stance when you consider that a 2013 issue of the *Journal of Patient Safety* released a study that concluded medical errors are the third leading cause of death in the United States (after heart disease and cancer). By contrast, Source energy is the *only* known cause of life.

When we speak of *Source energy*, we are speaking of that ultimate, creative force behind the birth and continuation of the *entire* cosmos, which flows throughout both the seen and unseen realms. The same great energy supply provided you with the body you currently inhabit and causes pine trees, aspens, rosebushes, cornstalks, and grasses to push through the earth's soils all across the planet, every day. In fact, the same energy is responsible for each form of life that has ever existed, past, present, and to come — *everywhere* — on our planet and all others.

Before we continue, let's pause for just a moment and reflect on the immensity of the Energy that created the universe as we know it, here on earth, even from our limited human perspective.

Scientists tell us the cosmos began billions of years ago as a tiny point, which was probably so small it would not have been detectable to the naked eye. This speck of unimaginable potential then exploded and began expanding with such force that, a fraction of one second into its newborn existence, it ballooned beyond the size of our own solar system. No more than an instant later, it dwarfed the entire Milky Way galaxy, giving birth to hundreds of billions of galaxies, each of which contained hundreds of billions of stars, whirling planets and their orbiting moons, flaming interstellar comets, and life in uncountable forms as it continued its mammoth expansion.

And it is still growing, even today, billions of years after its birth...

Now consider one more thing: it also gave birth to *you*. Your soul, your body, even your ego, all are a part of this fantastic, unfathomable birth. Do you really believe your doctor and a magic pill have the ability to understand your needs and heal your body better than the great Creator of the universe? What would make you think so? What causes so many of us to form such a curious impression? Do the doctors and pharmaceutical companies of the world somehow understand your body and what it needs to heal better than the force that created it, and sustains it every day, even now?

This is not meant to belittle those in the medical profession nor to discount their contributions to the realm of healing. But these are important questions we are wise to consider. Human beings are innately prone to making baseless assumptions about things we do not understand and have not considered with due care. This tendency not only limits us; in certain circumstances, it can be directly harmful.

When you align yourself — mind, body, and heart — with this immeasurably powerful Source, distress of any kind becomes impossible. This may sound too extreme to be true, and some might argue that it *cannot* be true due to the inevitable decline of physical life. That is to say, we all get sick, and we all, eventually, "die." True enough. But keep in mind that the body isn't the seat of life or the Source of its own healing. When you are absolutely in alignment with God, the body's atrophy will still occur as it did before, and you still may fall ill from time to time, but the consciousness behind the body will no longer suffer. In the sacred space of God enlightenment, there is so little attachment to the body that the mind exists in a protected state far beyond physical circumstances.

Yet even sustained enlightenment is not necessary in order to initiate the healing process. You do not have to become a saint in order to heal. The experience of God illumination is so powerful that just one instant in its presence can be enough to trigger a healing response.

When you are attempting to heal the body, then, you must focus on ridding yourself of the interference between you and the signal that Source broadcasts continually throughout the entire collective of life. Think of how a cell phone works. If you have ever tried having a phone conversation while inside a building with a metal roof, you already understand the trouble. Certain materials interfere with cell phones, causing poor reception. Interference with Source energy occurs in a similar way.

The seeds of sickness fester in those areas of your life where the interference with Source energy is greatest. These always occur at the human level. Your core Self exists in a state of immutability, and so it is forever healthy, protected, and safe because it is a direct and perfect extension of its Source. It needs no healing or defense of any kind. Your core Self can never be attacked, threatened, or made ill in any way, by any force or means, human or otherwise. There is no disease that can sicken it, no bullet that can wound it, no storm that can topple its walls. This part of you is immune to sickness, depression, fear, all forms of worldly ravages, and change of any kind. Your core Self was around before your body was born, and it will still be around after your body is no longer a functioning component of the earth.

Total healing can arise only through reconnecting with this ageless aspect of yourself — the original spark of life — in full awareness. You are in need of no other healing rituals beyond this. Your body itself is but a shadow of this ancient Being who dwells deep within you. In order for healing to come about, you must release all those things that contribute to disease by dampening this connection, and thus you open the channel that lets natural healing shine through.

In this sense, healing is actually a process of *releasing* the things that contribute to disease by blocking this experience, rather than adding a "healing agent" such as a physical remedy. For precisely this same reason, these interfering factors must be identified and undone, for it is only these that hold healing off and make it difficult. Systematically rooting out the forms of this opposition represents the real work of healing, and these are invariably emotional debris from the patient's past, like unhealed judgments, fear, guilt, old wounds, hatred, and various other malicious mental images and thoughts. In short, for healing to happen, the patient's heart must be cleansed of fear thoughts. Thus the journey of healing is truly a journey of purification.

The Healing Dimension

For our purposes we will refer to the experience of union with Spirit as "the healing dimension," which is a sort of *melting away* of the barriers that appear to separate you from other people and from Source. These barriers are actually not there and never really existed to begin with. This is another thing you learn when you come into contact with the presence of Source — the walls that appear to separate us exist only in our own minds, held in place by a lack of willingness to unite with others and the world around us in peace or, more accurately, to recognize the unity that is already there behind the appearance of division. This resistance to unity is the real force that keeps all seemingly separate haunts of the universe apart, and sickness intact as a result, for disease festers and grows only in the spaces that appear to separate us, just as bacteria only proliferates at certain temperatures.

During true healing, for a moment all sense of boundaries between you and another disappear, and you enter into a timeless space in which you cannot tell the difference between you and the other, nor would you choose to interfere with or disrupt the experience in any way. You simply let it be. Through this union you also recognize your oneness with Source, for unity with others *is* unity with Source, because each of us, at our Core, contains a perfect reflection of That which created us.

Of course, in time the doorway into this healing dimension will seem to close again, thus splitting off two who once knew their true, undivided divinity together, but this does not matter in the long term. Once this union occurs, healing has found a home in both patient and healer alike.

This sacred embrace has been experienced by many people, from every culture and every age, from all religions and no religion, and like Chi it has been called by many names: revelation, the mystical experience, samadhi, the holy instant, the healing dimension, and others. These are all different names for the same phenomenon. Whatever you choose to call it, it usually appears to arise spontaneously, with no obvious action or outward invitation needed on your part. However, if you look more carefully, you will realize that it still must be invited by the recipients on some level, otherwise it cannot be received. Just as healing cannot be forced on anyone, so too must this state be welcomed.

Entering the healing dimension involves a complete willingness to let go of all sense of a limited self, ego, awareness of the body, and even time and one's connection to the earthly existence itself. It is a state of total surrender. Granted, this vision requires only a temporary leave from ego existence, but for the interval in which it comes, you must become actively willing to step outside of time and space and know yourself as the formless, ageless, and eternal being you really are.

The healing dimension is usually experienced as a sudden shift away from the bodily level and a simultaneous merging into something greater. You may feel as if you are dissolving on one level, while awakening into the massive awareness of Source on another. There is no way to describe it, but we can say that it is generally accompanied by a deep sense of stillness, peace, and an exhilarating joy unimaginable from an ego-centered perspective. In the great formless state, there are no boundaries or limitations of any kind. This is precisely how it becomes possible to heal diseases without regard to the laws of medicine and physiology.

The soul emerging into this awareness for the first time may find it quite confusing and perhaps even startling, but once you are able to rise above any unsettled fear and relax, you will quickly adapt and understand the message revelation contains, which is a lesson in absolute freedom and boundless creation.

Though it may be difficult to accept at times, wellness is the natural state of the body. In this world, disease and death seem to be the normal course of the body as it ages. Obviously bodily existence is only a temporary experience. The body is a thing of time and earth, and as such it will not last forever, no matter how carefully you "guard your thoughts." The purpose of this book is not to teach physical immortality. There will come a time when each soul has learned all it can through its current lifetime and circumstances. Yet death need not be a thing that is thrust upon you as the result of some devastating illness that whisks you into oblivion, tearing you from the arms of your loved ones and seeming to end your life in a fit of fear and pain. Death can be a gentle process of letting go and being lifted free of the body, which is a lovely release that leads to joy and freedom. Yet to have this experience, the mind must be prepared to release the body without fear. This transition is an awakening to a different vision of life, not a retreat into the sleeping oblivion of death, which is all the common form of death truly is. A number of traditions and peoples have observed this, referring to death as "the great sleep," and similar terms. Consciously leaving the earth and awakening, instead of dying, is a choice everyone can make.

Assuming the patient wishes to heal and remain on earth for further learning, it must be understood that the healing process begins on the inside and works its way outward. The sequence proceeds from Source to core Self to the individual mind, and lastly into the body. You cannot reverse this order and hope to achieve a lasting solution. Furthermore, the steps involving Source and core Self are not our concern. Source forever radiates love, and core Self forever receives that love. The problem lies on the receiving end, within the mental framework of the individual. The nature of Chi is love, gentleness, and openness, but it can be said that the sick and suffering have fallen out of love with life; on some level it must be so.

Perhaps you believe that the body is rigid, inflexible, and cannot change, but it is really the mind that resists change. And it is *you*, the consciousness behind the body and mind both, that has the ultimate power to heal *both*. For you *can* change your thoughts. It is only a decision to do so, made with absolute conviction, that seems to separate you from a completely different vision of the body, through which you may recognize the body's littleness and Spirit's greatness.

Entering the Healing Dimension

While the experience of entering the healing dimension cannot be forced, it is highly useful to practice its mechanics. This process helps to open the mind and gradually steers it in the correct direction, lessening fear and increasing your desire to have the experience, which are the keys to its attainment.

You can practice entering this state simply by learning to become aware of the present, by releasing thoughts of the past and future, and turning inward, away from the outside world and toward the true seat of life — your core Self. It is helpful to practice entering this space regularly, regardless of whether or not you are sick, because the process also helps *maintain* a state of emotional balance and physical health. It is the key to living a healthier, happier life, and I believe it represents the ultimate evolutionary direction of life.

The more often you use the following meditation, the better you will get at it. Try it any time you experience fear, anxiety, depression, guilt, anger, or other turbulent emotions, as well as when you are already feeling quiet and at peace. It can be practiced anywhere, at any time, but whenever possible it is helpful to sit down and close your eyes. Minimally, you should aim to practice at least twice a day for five minutes or more, but if you find the exercise enjoyable, try using it occasionally throughout the day for longer periods of time.

Meditation on the Present Moment

1. Take a few deep breaths, inhaling through your nose and exhaling through your mouth. These do not have to be exaggerated breaths, but make sure you inhale slowly, fully, and most important, consciously, allowing air to fill the lower lobes of your lungs enough to cause your belly to rise, and exhaling in a similar fashion until all of the air is expelled. This process will begin tuning you in to the immediate sensations that can be felt in the body, and it instantly helps ease anxiety and draw you into the present.

2. Now, allow your breathing to return to normal and consciously let every muscle in your body relax (to whatever extent is practical depending on where you are). Spend a minute or more seeing how relaxed you can become. Try to sense any tension stored in your muscles dissipating, as if it is dispersing into the air. Start with your toes, feet, and legs, and work your way upward one muscle at a time.

3. When you are relaxed, focus on the sensation of air as it passes in and out of your nose. Concentrate on the spot where you feel the air first. This may be on your upper lip or at the tip of your nostrils. Notice how the air feels cooler as it enters your body, and warmer as it exits. Do not try to think about anything in particular. Just focus on the sensation of the air passing into and out of your body.

4. Keep your awareness on this process, feeling it directly. Try not to get caught up in thinking about the future or the past while you do this. For the purposes of this exercise, the only time that matters is right now — the *immediate moment*. Imagine that nothing else exists, no future and no past.

5. As thoughts do occur, instead of trying to resist them imagine that they are like clouds crossing the sky one by one, coming and going and shifting and vanishing as you watch them.

They are not you, and you are not them; they are passing images and words, and nothing more. When you do get caught up in some inner dialogue (which you *will*) remember to return your attention to the sense of air entering and exiting your body.

If you are doing this exercise correctly, you should experience a state of deepening restfulness, and you may feel a sense of spaciousness, openness, lightness, and a quiet joy. Allow this sensation to envelope you fully, and relax into it. Try to feel as if you are actually sinking into it, or as if it is enveloping you in a warm cocoon. The more you relax and let go, the closer you will come to connecting with the healing dimension. This exercise is so powerful that much healing can be achieved even at its shallowest levels.

CHAPTER FOUR

Into the Desert of Fear

Jordan's first round of chemo went well, or so it seemed. Based on the horror stories I'd heard regarding this particular class of drugs, I had expected him to be weaker and sicker than ever after treatment, but I was surprised when just the opposite occurred: he got some of his color back right away, his lymph nodes shrunk noticeably, and his energy increased. He was finally up and out of bed, and he even roused enough strength to hit the slopes with his brother and some friends for a morning of snowboarding.

Naturally we all took this as a good sign, an omen of things to come, and our hearts lightened, cautious smiles returning to weary faces across the board. For the moment, at least, a measure of our fear abated.

Yet there are many mirages along the path of disease. Like walking across a vast desert, staring into the distance plays tricks on the eyes. A shimmering of heat radiating from the desert floor gives rise to the illusion of a lake filled with life-sustaining water; a patterning of rocks at the horizon takes on the appearance of a forest of lush, green trees; and a bump in the terrain becomes a cabin.

As previously noted, when healing is not total, an illness is bound to resurface. This is so important, and indeed so astonishingly difficult to accept, that it needs significant reinforcement. Whether a disease shifts its outward face or comes again in its original form is irrelevant to the ultimate course of the patient. Such "healings" may provide a brief abatement of suffering, which, it can be argued, is a worthwhile accomplishment, allowing for a momentary respite from pain. However, with true healing being a possibility for the patient, it is clearly wiser to focus one's efforts on measures aimed at removing the deeper cause of the distress, as opposed to treatments that are destined to fail. Just like plucking weeds from a garden, you must be sure to pull up the root or you are merely wasting your efforts. Given time and the proper conditions, the weeds will all grow right back again.

Alas, it was not long before Jordan relapsed, an ominous sign that indicated the seriousness of his disease. It isn't that his doctor, or any of us for that matter, expected this first round of drugs to successfully treat Jordan's lymphoma. Chemotherapy generally requires a number of doses to fully rid the body of cancer. What was worrisome was the rapidity with which his symptoms returned. It was expected that he would remain free of major symptoms until his next dose of chemotherapy, or close to it, which was scheduled for some weeks later. Thus, though he at first responded well, the treatment was technically considered a failure. The unexpected, not to mention aggressive, return of his symptoms so quickly was akin to a desert traveler, actively dying of thirst, suddenly realizing that what he had taken to be a lake in the distance was merely more parched earth — dead, desolate, and just as sun-baked as the rest of the landscape.

As our newly born smiles dissolved, we little realized we had just boarded the emotional roller coaster of disease, with its soaring highs, sweeping lows, and blinding corners threatening to hurl us to our doom at any instant. Indeed, cancer is a vicious and wrenching ride, as are many serious illnesses. Real roller coasters would quickly lose their appeal if lives were at stake and if they went on and on, carrying everyone onboard for a terrifying journey through helplessness and fear, all the while promising no certain outcome. With cancer there isn't always a clear ending to the ride, one where the train slows and pulls into its little depot, squeals to a stop, and the safety bars lift, freeing passengers to disembark.

This is why it is of utmost importance for everyone involved in a patient's struggle to learn the art of seeking the calm of the present moment, instead of focusing on the mirages of hope that always seem to linger in the distance. True healing, as well as simple peace of mind, is a therapy the patient and his or her support network need to uncover within themselves by seeking the shelter of the here and now. Neither peace nor healing can be found by staring off into the horizon of the future, which presents mere phantom hopes for recovery and peace that are no more substantial than shifting desert mirages. Even when one does heal, it always happens in the present. It is only the *belief* that healing takes time to accomplish that delays its acceptance and subsequent manifestation into a patient's life. Alien as it may sound, to heal actually requires no time at all because it stems from the experience of going *beyond* time and into the healing dimension, which is a state that can only be accessed through the doorway of the eternal now.

Also, it is important to understand that the present extends more than just physical healing to those in need. During illness, whether you are the one undergoing treatment or are supporting someone else, the present is like the eye of a hurricane. It offers a space of calm and clarity at the storm's center, which is always accessible. There is no instant or circumstance in which the present is sealed off from you or anyone else. The moment you turn toward it — even just a little — you will experience some level of peace and abatement of symptoms.

This is why I encourage you to work regularly with the meditation in the previous chapter in order to experience just how powerful, certain, and yet gentle a protector the now really is. This is something that cannot be conveyed by words. I can describe the majesty, beauty, and omnipotence contained in the healing dimension, but no description will ever match the reality of the experience. While words can express its energy, it cannot be transmitted directly through human language. Only by experiencing it for ourselves can we understand, though it's an understanding that utilizes neither words, nor sounds, nor any symbolism at all.

This doesn't mean regular practice will completely shield you from stress and fear. While it is not my purpose to argue for our limitations, few living beings in this world have reached a level of perfect serenity in which they remain completely liberated from fear all the time. I have been told it is possible to reach such a state, but not having personally attained it, I cannot testify directly. In fact, when Jordan relapsed I was instantly jarred into a deep fear state and hurled from the present moment uncontrollably as if against my own will. It was a humbling reminder of my own imperfect mastery of present-moment awareness.

At this point in his treatment Jordan's physician decided to take an aggressive step. Dr. Martin admitted Jordan to the hospital so that he could be closely monitored during an intensive, five-day chemotherapy regimen. Hospitalization was necessary due to the dangerous nature of this treatment, as Jordan's body would be receiving a significant dose of what amounted to poison, and his immune system would be severely compromised. In other words, the "medication" might kill him!

As it turned out, the treatment did not kill him, but it didn't seem to help much either. While the symptoms of his lymphoma moderately retreated at first, by the time he checked out of the hospital afterward, he looked weaker, sicker, and more withdrawn than ever. We assumed that the chemotherapy had caused his deteriorated condition and that, as he recovered, his health would improve. We were soon to discover, however, that making assumptions is a tricky, and very often disappointing, venture when it comes to cancer.

Although medicine is exploring a number of promising new therapies to treat cancers, as of this writing there are still only four major, widely accepted ways to deal with it: chemotherapy, radiation therapy, surgery, and stem-cell transplants. During chemotherapy, the cancer is essentially poisoned with chemicals in an attempt to rid the body of the dysfunctional cells; radiation therapy aims to zap the cancer growth into oblivion with focused doses of high energy particles or waves; and surgery attempts to remove cancer the old-fashioned way, by incising it from the body. (Later, we will discuss stem-cell transplants in more detail, as these are more complicated, and we'll describe targeted therapies as well, which are basically a form of "smart chemo.") Unfortunately, by the time Jordan was diagnosed, his cancer had already progressed too far to treat with radiation, and surgery is not a standalone option for most lymphomas.

It was not long before we realized that the aggressive treatment had clearly failed to stop Jordan's lymphoma. Just as he was recovering from the walloping side effects of his second round of chemo, he sank into disease yet again, his symptoms raging, lymph nodes swollen and badly painful.

On an interesting side note, the worsening of Jordan's symptoms typically coincided with various interpersonal conflicts. It was clear that these conflicts were in part triggered by the stress of the illness itself, but they consistently caused flare-ups in his condition — a vicious, self-perpetuating cycle that became clearer to me as his treatments progressed, and which convinced me that his disease was wildly responsive to his mental state. As this cycle became apparent, I began counseling Jordan on the role the mind plays in healing, and I led him through visualization and meditation exercises, casually at first but with increasing depth as his disease progressed. I admit, this was a topic I had previously been hesitant to broach with Jordan, mainly due to his age. I had wrongly assumed that he wouldn't be interested in meditation and mind-body philosophies of healing. As it turned out, Jordan showed genuine interest, and he proved to be a natural at meditation, which goes to show how foolish and warped our own perceptions can be.

While I worked to uncover the root of Jordan's illness, a third chemo treatment was devised and administered, this one using yet another cocktail of chemo drugs called Gemzar. One of the problems with chemotherapy is that some cancers are able to adapt to specific drugs before the patient is cured, in a manner resembling how bacteria may overcome a particular antibiotic. Once adaptation occurs, the drug becomes far less effective, or even useless, making it necessary to try something else. With Jordan's condition deteriorating daily and his lymph nodes swollen in various locations throughout his body, causing terrible pain as well as constant enervation, his situation shifted from one of hope and optimism to a sense of real emergency. If this next treatment also failed, it might indicate that *all* standard chemo options were off the table.

To his credit, Dr. Martin didn't wait to see what Jordan's response to the Gemzar would be. He began making phone calls right away to major medical centers around the country that specialized in Jordan's particular form of aggressive lymphoma, fishing for alternative treatments. He seemed to already know what the rest of us could only guess at: Jordan needed options, and he needed them immediately.

This moment of urgency also marked a turning point for me personally. Around this time I became aware of one other concern that had been chipping away at my peace of mind, though I had apparently relegated it into unconsciousness. I realized that I wasn't concerned exclusively with Jordan's well-being. I was terrified for my daughter as well. Brittany carries a beautiful light within her. She is a gorgeous being, inside and out, and the thought of her having to watch her boyfriend, whom she clearly loved, die a horrendous and painful death at such a young age was unbearable for me. As Jordan's disease progressed, terrifying images began bombarding me day and night, invading even my ordinarily peaceful dreams. For a time, there seemed no escaping them, no relief from the hell of my imagination.

Another curious thought occurred to me around this time, which my mind got stuck in like sneakers in freshly laid tar. During the summer before Jordan fell ill, three tourists with a church group were visiting Yosemite National Park in California when they were swept over Vernal Falls to their deaths. The Merced River was running at record levels that year as the result of massive snowfall, causing this particular waterfall to become a raging beast.

When I was a child, my father took my siblings and me camping in Yosemite many times, and I hiked to the top of Vernal Falls during each visit. It was my favorite hike, leading trekkers up and along a treacherous, often slick, series of steps to the top of a most spectacular vision. In full bloom, Vernal Falls presents one of the most majestic natural sights along the West Coast. It is 317 feet high and plunges into a boulder-strewn chute at its base. The trail up is aptly known as the Mist Trail because when the falls are in full fury, hikers get blasted by water vapor all the way to the top, which is a refreshing and exhilarating experience on a hot summer afternoon.

As a kid I recall standing near the brink of the falls during one particular summer trip when the river was flowing at peak levels. The spectacle was awesome and equally terrifying. Signs were posted everywhere admonishing visitors to stay clear of the river's edge and warning of the powerful current and slippery rocks — a hazardous combination to be sure.

On July 20, 2011, two visitors apparently ignored this warning. A girl not much older than Brittany decided to wade out into the river a short way upstream from the waterfall in order to reach a small isle that somehow manages to survive, year after year, precariously perched only twenty or thirty feet from the crest of the falls. A guy from her group accompanied her.

I know this island well. It is indeed a spectacle. As a child I imagined that if I ever fell into the river by accident I would swim for it in a last-ditch attempt at survival. When the river is really low, one can safely walk out to it, and I can understand the temptation to want to reach it. Thankfully, I was never foolish enough to try.

The girl and her companion did not make it. A short way out, the water raging around their knees, they slipped and were instantly swept into the full thrust of the current. A third guy from their group reportedly tried to grab hold of them in a feeble rescue attempt, lost his balance, and was also whisked away.

Dozens of people witnessed this tragedy. According to accounts, the first pair clung to each other as they were launched over the waterfall, and one witness, who was standing just above the brink, told reporters that he locked eyes with the third victim as the man vanished over the cusp in silence and plummeted to his death. The witness said it was the most horrible experience of his life, and he felt he'd been permanently scarred by the terror and shock inscribed on the man's face, which seared itself into his memory.

For some reason I became temporarily obsessed with this incident while Jordan was going through his ordeal months later. I kept imagining it in vivid detail in my mind's eye. Despite my horror, I could find no way to stop the visions from bombarding me. It became a visceral experience that almost felt *real* at times, as if I had actually been there and witnessed the accident myself.

My childhood memories of standing at the edge of Vernal Falls dominated my thoughts, lending grisly details to my imagination as I observed, in my mind's eye, these three youths racing along the river's current to their doom. Morbid as it sounds, I wondered what they thought: What did they feel as they began their plummet and gravity took hold of their destiny? What did they see? Did they close their eyes, or did they watch?

It took me some time to realize what my strange obsession was really about, but eventually I came to understand that Jordan's predicament felt to my subconscious mind much like we were being swept toward the precipice of a waterfall, and there was nothing anyone could do to help — not for all the doctors, medications, and money in the world. All anyone could do was stand by and passively watch. And the treatments Jordan was receiving seemed a lot like that island in the center of the river, perched above the falls. Alluring and promising as the island appeared from the river's edge, it was fully unreachable and represented nothing more than a mirage of hope. We were all in the current together, and a waterfall was dead ahead.

PART TWO

Special Principles of Healing

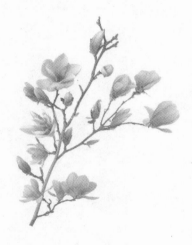

Our life is shaped by our mind, for we become what we think.
Suffering follows an evil thought
as the wheels of a cart follow the oxen that draw it.

— BUDDHA

CHAPTER FIVE

The Patient Must Believe
Healing Is Possible

The Special Principles of Healing are critical to the healing process. In truth, they are so important they might be
thought of as "laws of healing." They are not laws in the traditional sense. There are no Cosmic police officers who enforce
them, charges to be answered, sentences to be served. Rather, the
Special Principles are based on simple cause-and-effect relationships that exist between thoughts, emotions, and the body. There
is no magic behind them. They are, in effect, merely statements
similar to the laws of physics. They do not judge you or your
situation any more than gravity does. If you fall from a tree, gravity will propel you toward the earth. This doesn't mean you will
necessarily be injured or hit the ground. Perhaps you'll catch a
limb on the way down or land softly in a bush. The law of gravity
simply dictates that all matter within Earth's gravitational field is
drawn toward the planet's mass. Likewise the Special Principles
are simple, always in effect, and completely neutral.

On a practical level, think of these as guidelines that can help
you align, and then stay aligned, with a state of wellness on every

plane of your being. The Special Principles might also be considered conditions that every patient must meet in order to heal at the deepest level of disease, no matter how major or minor an illness may be. This is not a punitive matter. As you will see, the power of these principles is the result of the sheer force of the patient's own will.

Special Principle of Healing 1

The patient must believe healing is possible.

This concept may seem elementary, and indeed it is, as are most of the ideas in this book. Our first Special Principle merely stems directly from the notion that the patient's mind is the primary component influencing health and healing. Special Principle 1, then, is really an extension of the basic Principles of Healing. However, it is important to understand that thoughts not only affect the body's condition in general; a patient's *beliefs* about whether or not recovery is even possible directly influence the healing outcome.

This means that if a patient believes he or she is going to recover, the person will make that outcome more likely through this belief. The patient's conviction does not have to be firm and unwavering by any means, but the overall vision must steer the person toward healing. Likewise, if a patient believes he or she will *not* get better, and this vision dominates the person's mind, an impediment to healing is created. As a result, the person's recovery is likely to be hampered at a fundamental level.

To jump ahead in Jordan's story for a moment, eventually his condition became critical, and Jordon was flown by plane from Bend to the Oregon Health & Science University Hospital in Portland, a major treatment center. After I arrived and joined Jordan in the ICU, I recognized right away that Special Principle 1 was being challenged in a major way, and I immediately set out to help him deal with it. Jordan was in a stunning, not to mention terrifying, situation: his room was full of doctors who were indicating, mostly through inference and behavior, that he was going to die. Any patient is apt to believe their doctors without question in this circumstance, especially a kid of Jordan's age. After all, they are the experts. They deal in disease and healing and death every day. It's the job they've trained for.

To be clear, Jordan's doctors didn't intend to undermine his determination to heal. Medical care professionals often find themselves in a quandary. Using all their knowledge and experience, they must be honest and clear with the patient about his or her prognosis as they view it. If the patient has little chance of recovery, a physician is required by law to say so, and eventually they said so to Jordan. This carries a great responsibility, however. Many a patient has been overcome by disease only because it seemed easier to give up, instead of continuing to fight on though there was no apparent hope of getting better. In the midst of suffering, it may indeed feel easier just to let go and vanish, albeit temporarily, into "the great sleep." This temptation is often present during severe illness, and it only gets worse if the patient cannot see the proverbial light at the end of the tunnel.

If a doctor tells a patient that he or she is going to die, and the patient believes the doctor, it becomes more likely to happen. This is a very simple yet profound phenomenon, and all medical professionals need to be aware of it. If they are to perform their jobs with optimal proficiency, they must become actively aware that their foremost responsibility is to promote health through love, hope, and the joy of living — all while finding a way to communicate clearly and honestly with patients and their families. This is a challenge, and no doubt it is a skill that many doctors do not learn much about while attending medical school. Nevertheless, it is their most vital asset. They may have learned the mechanics of the body and the chemistry of pills, and learned them well, yet the truth remains unalterable: illness is a *spiritual* crisis. To treat the body is fine, but to treat it *exclusively* is a meaningless endeavor.

This is why when all hope seemed lost in Jordan's case, I knew it was of urgent importance to rekindle it. Immediately after I arrived at the hospital in Portland, I identified the unfolding situation for what it was, even though Jordan and the doctors were still waiting for the test results that would confirm what no one yet wanted to voice out loud. Jordan seemed to realize it, too: his eyes were hollow with the fear of death, and he looked thoroughly hopeless and lost, despite the fact that Jordan, by nature, is one of the most courageous people I've ever known. It was a terrible moment to witness, and death was palpable in the room. It is a hard feeling to describe to those who have never experienced it, but impending death is something that can be sensed. Years before, I'd felt the same sensation in the room with my mother shortly before her death. There are many accounts of this phenomenon.

The first thing I did was to sit down at Jordan's bedside, look him directly in the eyes, and tell him the following words, which felt to me like both the most difficult, and at the same time enlightened, words I had ever spoken. I said, "Jordan, no matter what these people tell you, no matter what is to come, no matter what the doctors say, there is one thing I want you to remember: *with love, all things can be healed.*"

Perhaps it may seem that this little speech should have been of negligible help in such dire circumstances, especially when held up against what the doctors were about to tell him. Indeed, I am inclined to agree. After all, the important part consisted of only seven words. Why should Jordan believe what I was saying when the doctors were telling him something completely different? Looking back, I am honestly not sure I fully understand the answer myself, but the one thing I did feel was that the words I spoke were not words that came *from* me, Tobin Blake, the writer, the meditation teacher, the ego, the man. They were words that came *through* me, from God, and they contained a seed of healing that I alone could never plant.

However it happened, something within Jordan clicked and aligned with the words, despite what the doctors were predicting, and somehow through his distress he grasped the kernel of hope they held out to him. He took them in and made them a part of his own thoughts and heart. Then he accomplished something most remarkable — he proved them to be true.

Awakening Hope

Because the patient must believe healing is possible in order to recover, a vital early step in the healing process is awakening, or reinforcing, hope. Even if doctors predict that healing is not possible — either because the disease is deemed terminal or because it's simply incurable, if not necessarily fatal — the patient needs to hear directly, clearly, and with conviction that healing is *always* possible. This does not mean you should become confrontational with the person or the medical professionals involved. Keep in mind that some patients are highly resistant to the notion that they can heal, and creating conflict during an already challenging time never helps.

If anyone involved in a medical situation resists the healing principles and techniques presented in this book, don't argue or try to force them to agree. Instead, remain focused on gently encouraging the patient to keep an open mind, and be supportive of every effort he or she makes to recover.

However, when people *are* open minded to alternative healing therapies and ideas, but they have been told that healing is not possible, consider sharing these key points:

- Regardless of what the patient has been told, remember that doctors are not God. They cannot see the future of any given individual. When they diagnose a patient, they are merely stating their opinion, and doctors have been wrong countless times. This is a fact.
- There are many verifiable cases of spontaneous healing, and if something is possible for any one of us, it must be possible for *all* of us. Such unexplained cases should remind us of our own potential for healing, just as Roger Bannister proved that the four-minute-barrier was an imaginary limitation. Illusions of the limits of healing can, and should, be risen above.
- We are spiritual beings having a human experience, not the other way around. The body is not inflexible. It will change and heal as the mind changes and heals.
- The body is naturally drawn toward health and healing, and, in reality, it is a phenomenal healing instrument. Health only requires the right conditions and, most important, the appropriate mind-set. Disease, on the other hand, is an unnatural state and will dissipate when the conditions that caused it are no longer present.
- In regards to physical treatments, medical science is rapidly evolving new treatments all the time. A disease that is supposedly incurable today may be readily treatable tomorrow. This is not an exaggeration. Medicine and our understanding of the human body are expanding at a historically unprecedented rate.
- Finally, it is vital to remember that life is the ultimate force of the universe. Life is, literally, the will of God. Where life is possible, it will flourish. And where there is life, there is always a way.

Most of all, inspire the patient through your own sense of hope, love, and joy for life. These forces are more convincing than any words could ever hope to be because they are an extension of your own will and love for life. Thus they inspire through example, and by doing so they hold the power to infuse the patient with the raw desire to live, which is without a doubt the most potent healing elixir of all.

CHAPTER SIX

The Patient Must Want to Heal

At first glance it may sound ridiculous to suggest that in order to heal the patient must *want* to heal. Of course the patient wants to heal! Don't they? After all, who in their right mind would not wish to be healthy, happy, and at peace if the choice was theirs to make?

Yet this is precisely the problem with sickness. It creates a state of what might be called *non-right-mindedness*, and it is from this state that disease is conceived, nourished, and preserved from healing by the oblivion of unconsciousness. Principle of Healing 6 (page 41) touched on this notion, but it needs to be examined in more detail to be fully understood and, ultimately, undone.

Special Principle of Healing 2
The patient must want to heal.

In this section we come to one of the greatest hurdles to healing that every patient faces. It is a step that requires tremendous courage and unflinching honesty to conquer, for in this step patients must confront their own unconscious darkness, fears, sense of guilt, the wish to do harm to others, as well as the wish to *be hurt* in return. To surmount this particular obstacle to healing, patients must seek to uproot *every* hidden motivation in their unconscious and conscious mind to side with suffering.

As discussed previously, sickness almost never *seems* to be a decision. I have had the experience myself on numerous occasions when I've become ill and been told by my inner Teacher — in one form or another — that I've done this to myself. *A Course in Miracles* teaches, "Sickness is not an accident.... [It] is a decision. It is not a thing that happens to you, quite unsought.... It is a choice you make, a plan you lay." What an exceedingly annoying thing to say to a sick person! Most, if not all, patients are bound to resist the notion at first, to resent it, to question and doubt it, and at times to actively quarrel with it or dismiss it outright. You might wonder, *Why would I wish illness upon myself?* It is indeed an important question to consider. I have asked it of myself many times, in many forms, and on each occasion the first response that came to mind was something like, *If I did choose this miserable experience, I certainly don't remember doing so.*

Here, then, is the great hurdle to aligning with Special Principle 2. It isn't that it is a difficult concept to understand intellectually. Rather, the real challenge lies in attempting to discover one's own darkness hidden in the inner mind, for the theory as taught by *A Course in Miracles* goes on to suggest that sickness is a decision that is made *and then forgotten about* and buried in unconsciousness. This is why illness does not appear to be a choice, but something that just suddenly occurs without our invitation. Furthermore, the theory holds, this choice is not made in a vacuum; it serves a *purpose*. In other words, the decision is made in order to achieve some desired outcome; we choose disease for a *reason*, to give us something we believe we want.

I admit, this may sound absurd, but the further I have gone along my own spiritual path, which *is* what the path of healing really is, the more convinced I have become that, despite how infuriating the idea can be at times (not to mention insulting, frustrating, and a few other things!), it is fundamentally true.

With that in mind, I urge you to find a way to welcome this idea and make it a part of your own healing arsenal, regardless of any resistance your ego may feel toward it. Remember that the ego, by definition, is a false self, which means it is bound to feel threatened by your true Self, which represents your reality. In turn the ego wants *you* to feel threatened so that you will stay identified with it and unable to see beyond its narrow existence to what you really are. This is the only state in which the ego feels safe. Therefore any idea that reminds you of your Divine nature and the boundless power that exists within you, beyond the ego's limitations, makes the ego feel particularly vulnerable.

This is the real reason many people lash out against the idea that sickness is a design of the mind, not because they loathe the suggestion that they are responsible for their own suffering. Egos hate any idea that reminds us that our survival is not dependent on either the ego or the body. Of itself, the notion that we are in command of our health and, ultimately, our own destiny is clearly not inherently offensive. Why would it be? On the contrary, it is liberating and empowering. What you leave behind when you accept this idea is weakness, fear, and the belief in a random, chaotic universe; what you gain is a sense of strength and safety that comes from the realization of the universe's true nature, which is a place of order, care, and all-encompassing Divine love.

Harnessing Special Principle 2

Once the patient begins to accept — if not embrace — the notion that disease starts as a decision, which like all decisions is made by the mind, the second stage of aligning with Special Principle 2 is to seek out and understand what purpose you are attempting to use sickness for. How is it serving you?

Does this not follow naturally? What good is it to learn that sickness is a decision with a purpose if you do not then seek to uncover what that purpose must be? Once you understand the reason behind your choice, you then become free to *change your mind* and move in another, more positive direction. This is how healing is brought about, and as challenging as it can be in its application, the process actually has only three simple steps:

1. Realize sickness is a choice.
2. Figure out why you made that choice.
3. Make a different choice.

The motivations for choosing disease may be as varied as are individual personalities. However, most fit into just a few major categories. In general, the patient seeks some kind of reward or payoff through sickness. Therefore, the person must become deeply honest and look inward with unflinching resolve to seek and find the truth behind the all-important question:

"What am I getting out of this?"

Sickness for Attention

The tendency to use sickness in order to get attention typically forms early in life, oftentimes as an unintentional gift bequeathed from well-meaning adults. Perhaps when you were a child you received extra attention, and even "treats," from your parents or other people when you became ill. Wanting to care for our loved ones when they are sick is a normal reaction, and love does help the healing process. In this respect, the response cannot be said to be a bad thing in itself. The problem arises when a person develops a long-term pattern of attention-seeking through sickness.

As in all cases of disease, people are probably not aware they are doing this. Sickness just seems to happen to them more often than to others. Also, in some instances these individuals may exhibit an increased tendency to engage in illness-inducing behaviors, like overeating, not exercising, smoking, and engaging in various other self-destructive activities. In such cases these negative behavioral choices are usually only a device designed to realize the patient's unconscious desire to be ill. In this sense they are similar in basic function to healing instruments — such as medications and other physical remedies — that seem to heal the body. Essentially these things and behaviors provide a form intended to make manifest that which is latent in the unconscious mind.

The personality type that exhibits this pattern of disease-seeking often craves attention but may feel regularly neglected or overlooked by, and perhaps less connected to, their primary friends and family. If you find yourself using sickness in order to get attention, the corrective solution lies, in part, in breaking the cycle by improving your relationships, particularly during periods of nonillness. It is helpful to intentionally, *consciously*, seek to improve your connection to others by making the effort to fearlessly foster the exchange of love in all of your relationships, learning to communicate openly and gently, and spending quality time with loved ones often.

Those stuck in this pattern may also find it useful to start thinking of themselves as a unique and glorious creation of the universe, which they are. You do not need illness to get attention, which will always leave you feeling empty. Nor is *attention*, per se, satisfying to the soul. What is satisfying is celebrating yourself for what you are, as you are. Strive to become an example of the perfection human beings are meant to be, and let your unique gifts shine for everyone to witness. In this way you will no longer feel the need for attention-seeking through illness. You will receive the purest and most meaningful attention any of us could hope to draw — the attention of your own true Self.

Sickness for Escape

Just as attention is one form of reward that sickness may bring, so too disease can offer an escape from the pressures of life. Once again, this is very often learned early as a child. Who hasn't faked an illness in order to play hooky from school? This is a simple reward-based behavior. When you get sick, you can justify taking the day off without feeling guilty about it.

This type of disease-seeking is not a significant issue if it occurs only rarely in its minor forms, but for some people it may become a lifelong pattern that can take on forms of serious, debilitating afflictions. This pattern may develop when an individual uses disease as a means to escape the normal interactions and responsibilities of society permanently or for long stretches of time. The major telling symptom is when someone develops a chronic, "incurable" illness that renders the person incapable of working or otherwise constructively contributing to their own welfare.

Once again, the answer to this form of disease-seeking is simple. In this case, the development of *passion* may provide an answer. Very often those who find themselves caught up in this pattern simply haven't determined what their true calling is, and so work, and life in general, ends up feeling empty, dull, and meaningless, which most jobs are. However, when pursued with determination, your true calling will satisfy you in ways that nothing else in the world can. When you follow your passion, you feel as if something within you just clicks into place, and you know — deep down in a way you never will be able to fully describe to others — that you have found your soul's gift to the world. Whatever it turns out to be, this work is what you were born to contribute, and that is why you will find it so deeply satisfying. Your being will ring with truth when you pursue it. Furthermore, by following your true calling with full dedication and trust, you will receive the support of the entire universe. This is a remarkable response, but also a predictable one. Perhaps you won't get rich from following your passion, but you will find that all your basic needs are met, somehow, someway, and the necessary doors to make your journey possible will open before you even reach them (that is, assuming you are willing to have them opened; as with healing, your willingness is a key ingredient to receiving Cosmic assistance).

Your true calling will typically feel so natural, and bring you such joy as it develops, that once you dedicate yourself to it, you may find yourself wanting to do little else. I rarely take a day off from writing because for me, writing is not really work. It is my "calling," or at least a part of it. I also use it as a form of "letting go, and letting God," to quote an old Christian saying, and a meditation on the present. I imagine I will continue to share my thoughts via the written word to the end of this physical incarnation, regardless of any worldly rewards or lack of them.

The point is, once you begin doing what Source has called you to do, you will be far less tempted to use sickness as a way to avoid work because, for you, there will be no work; Source will do the work for you and through you. This is what it means to serve God. All you will need to do is allow it to happen.

Sickness for Money

This motive hardly needs clarifying. Money is one of the driving incentives behind an overwhelming portion of human behavior, both in constructive as well as destructive versions. Desperate people may lie, cheat, steal, beg, and borrow themselves into financial ruin, and some people even commit murder in the name of money. It should come as little surprise, then, that some people use illness and injury as a way to obtain money.

Because of all the devious behavior associated with money, many people believe that money is evil, or at least that, as the saying goes, it is "the root of all evil." The truth, however, is that money is not evil. It is just a force, an idea of agreed-upon valuation, an energy system. Just like gravity, it is actually neutral. Money may be used for positive as well as negative agendas, depending on the individual's intent. Therefore the answer to the dilemma of money's misuse is not to rid the world of it, but to heal the head and heart of those who employ it — a population that includes each of us.

In order to heal any form of sickness that is caused by the drive for money, the patient needs to realize, fully and clearly, that money will never bring the happiness they crave, and this is a fact, not an opinion. David Geffen, the billionaire philanthropist and founder of Geffen Records, once succinctly put it this way: "Anybody who thinks money will make you happy, hasn't got money." Words don't get much clearer than that.

It is also interesting to note that many people who suddenly become rich have observed this same truth. In reality, with more money typically come more worries, and logic itself suggests that a miserable poor person who instantly becomes wealthy will likely simply become a miserable rich person. If happiness is the ultimate gauge for life satisfaction, what is the point?

I'd like to suggest something that you may find radical, but which I have come to believe in wholeheartedly. Let us, you and I, seek to be wise and listen to our fellow humans who have experienced what it is like to be rich and who have seen that more money leads to no lasting increase in joy. Once again, it isn't that money is evil; it's just that it won't make you happy. Yet rich or poor, happiness is indeed possible. But to have it, you must first set aside your belief and dreams that becoming wealthy will solve whatever emptiness you feel. It decidedly will not. What does satisfy, on the other hand, is the realization that the emptiness *is not there*. It only seems to exist while you seek for satisfaction through sources outside of yourself, since the quest for external satisfaction shifts your focus away from *what is satisfying*. Once you turn inward for satisfaction, and focus on the present moment, you find a deep and lasting sense of relief, with no waiting necessary. Your hope for future satisfaction can be resolved immediately.

Sickness for Self-Punishment

It may be hard to comprehend how punishment, in any form, could be something that is sought after, but in actuality internalized guilt is *the* major contributor to disease. When you feel guilty, you inevitably believe that you deserve to be punished. This is what guilt does. Like so many causal factors of disease, guilt and the corresponding urge it produces for punishment may not be something you are even aware of, but the drive eventually produces suffering on some level, in some form.

The way to escape this perverse cycle is to identify the things you feel most guilty about — a process that requires immense self-honesty — and then heal those things through *right action* and *right thought*. One solution may be dedicating yourself to healing any wrongs you may have committed. The key, however it comes about, is to find some way to forgive yourself for your mistakes. This may or may not involve the specific people or incidents that triggered the guilt. Let's use an extreme example to help understand this process: suppose one night a woman has a few drinks at a friend's house and gets involved in a car accident on her way home, taking the life of an innocent child. This would be an emotionally devastating trauma for anyone, and it would likely result in extreme feelings of guilt. How could this woman heal herself?

To begin with, it is necessary to accept the fact that we cannot change the past. We may as well come to peace with this right now, for it is true. The past is literally gone. We have no power over it whatsoever. To dwell on it is to weaken and deprive ourselves of the power we *do* have, which is the power to shape and change the future through our *present* decisions, thoughts, and actions.

For instance, in this extreme example, this woman might help heal her guilt by dedicating herself to ensuring that others do not make the same mistake she did. By acting in the present as a voice of awareness regarding the dangers of driving while intoxicated, she would work to save innocent lives in the future.

Whatever the situation, we can only amend mistakes using whatever means are immediately available. The present moment holds the key to this healing path, while the past itself, where the mistake occurred, is useless when it comes to repairing the present.

Of course, this is just an example of how one might seek to heal lingering guilt from a past error. In reality, no actions are necessary for forgiveness to be accepted. Making amends for past mistakes is merely one way of aiding the process of forgiving guilt. In this example, right action promotes a state of right-mindedness, from which physical recovery from guilt-induced illnesses is bound to follow.

Another important thing to clarify is that it isn't necessary for others to forgive you in order to be free of guilty feelings. The loved ones of a victim who was killed in a drunk driving accident may or may not choose to forgive the person who was at fault in the accident. Other people's forgiveness is not something we can control or force. All of us have our own lessons in Earth School that we were born to learn, and no one can dictate to another what those lessons are or when they should become open to learning them. What we are able to control is the timing behind *when* we choose to accept and learn our own life lessons.

Sickness for Attack

Just as suffering can be used as a tool to punish oneself, it can also be directed toward others. This system of attack is often aimed at those to whom the patient is closest, such as a romantic partner, parents, or the patient's own children, but it can be used to attack anyone, including total strangers.

While it is true that a patient may use illness in order to cause their loved ones fear, financial strain, and other difficulties, this is almost always little more than a surface objective. If you look deeper into the motivations behind this form of assault, guilt usually plays a leading role. The objective is to use illness to cause others to feel guilty. This may be a blatant maneuver, such as when a patient openly accuses others of causing, or at least contributing to, their disease, or it may be more subtle, as when an individual becomes ill and their close friends and family feel an underlying — and often unacknowledged — sense of guilt due to not being able to ease their suffering.

As when a patient uses sickness as self-punishment, some form of forgiveness is the primary remedy because forgiveness is the opposite of not only anger but guilt. Also note that guilt is actually anger directed inward, against oneself, and anger is guilt projected outward at the world. If you look carefully, you may notice that whenever you feel guilty, you simultaneously experience an impulse to purge yourself of it, since guilt is among the most vile and actively destructive of all human emotions. Anger is really nothing more than the attempt to displace guilt onto someone else by seeing them as more guilty than you are; in this way, you become less guilty or "innocent" by comparison. This is the "guilt cycle," which will be discussed in detail later.

In short, displacing guilt on others does not work for several reasons. For one thing, "less guilty" does not equate to "not guilty." Thus you still experience guilt. Second, the attempt to project guilt *never* actually works. Actually, it only *increases* your sense of guilt because you now feel additional guilt for becoming angry in the first place. This is true even when the anger remains unexpressed and internalized.

Forgiveness undoes this destructive cycle at a deep level. It is so effective that it could rightly be called God's own healing therapy. No guilt-driven disease can withstand true forgiveness. Therefore, for those patients who discover that they are using sickness as a weapon, forgiveness is your primary prescription. Take daily as needed, and call your spiritual counselor if the urge to attack persists.

Sickness and Drug Seeking

My wife is a nurse who spent years working in an emergency room, and this particular illness-inducing motive was something she saw all the time. Every age has its plagues, and drug addiction is one of the most destructive diseases ever to confront the human race. Whether we are speaking of pills, alcohol, or hard drugs, the effect of addiction can be ruinous on multiple levels of the patient's life — financially, socially, professionally, physically, and emotionally.

Addiction encourages disease in several ways. First of all and most obviously, excessive drug and alcohol abuse put a severe strain on the body, making disease more likely. Just as pertinent, however, is the fact that because drugs are usually controlled by our society, and addictions tend to be expensive, people often become desperate when they are unable to readily attain their drug of choice. Thus they may end up in the doctor's office — or quite commonly the ER — with an endless array of symptoms that require pain pills, antianxiety meds, muscle relaxants, and other forms of medication, which coincidentally produce intoxication.

Let me clarify here that this is not a lecture on the so-called evils of addiction. Alcoholism and drug addiction are diseases like any other, and once people get locked into an addiction cycle, it can be exceedingly challenging to overcome. Blame is as ridiculous in addiction cases as in any other disease. Likewise, the stance that addicts choose their state of dependence and therefore do not deserve compassion and understanding is equally unhelpful. As usual, blame does not solve the problem.

With that said, healing from addiction still involves lowering one's defenses and facing the true cause of the disease, difficult and unsavory as this process may at first feel. Facing truths and looking within ourselves with honesty opens us to a great power. When a patient goes to a doctor complaining of some symptoms, a wise physician doesn't immediately write prescriptions for every ache and pain the person describes. Instead, the doctor seeks to discover what is *causing* the symptoms. The reason is that treating symptoms without also addressing their cause is meaningless.

Likewise, the active denial of the real cause of a disease, or of any problem for that matter, is a common defense against healing, and it is a particularly prevalent defense in the drug addict's arsenal. Most addicts do not want their addiction addressed. They cannot see any hope for happiness beyond the high of their chosen drug. They don't realize that the addiction itself has robbed them of their ability to experience the natural joy inherent in life.

When an addict goes to the emergency room complaining of some pain for which they want medication, it's not that they are knowingly lying about their condition, although sometimes they certainly do. Very often they are in real pain. Whether or not a doctor feels that the pain is all in the person's "head" is really an irrelevant question. In one sense, *all* pain is in a patient's head, since the mind is the seat of consciousness and thus the ultimate interpreter of what is painful and what is pleasurable.

The solution to this grim situation is that the patient must develop a sense of happiness and joy beyond the addiction. Attempting to quit or stop what is addicting is not enough on its own, and in fact can cause deep depression and a sense of hopelessness, which is *never* helpful. It is wiser to cultivate a deepening awareness of the joy that comes from spiritual vision, which will automatically, and gradually, reduce the impulse to engage self-destructively. Paramahansa Yogananda once recommended that meditation students *not* give up sex, but instead meditate regularly and then compare the feelings meditative practice produces with those found during sexual activity. He knew the truth, which is simply that the state of deep meditation is far more gratifying than sex ever will be. Yet how can you convince someone of that who has never experienced deep meditation? You can't. You can only show them how to discover it for themselves.

Sickness for Death

Sometimes illness is brought about specifically for the purpose of death. Certainly, like pain, death is no reward, although those deluded into believing there is no joy possible in life may come to believe so, albeit unconsciously like so many of the motivations for disease. On a side note, death is not to be confused with the conscious, final exit of the body undertaken by enlightened beings who have finished their earthly lessons in their present incarnation. This is called *mahasamadhi* in Eastern religious traditions or "conscious death" in contemporary terms. Where death is a retreat into deep sleep, *mahasamadhi* can rightly be considered an awakening.

For those who have become disillusioned with life and have lost all sense of hope for happiness, death may come to be viewed as an escape from pain. This form of disease often arises as the result of highly distressing relationships and worldly circumstances that appear to have no possible resolution. When this occurs, hopelessness takes over, just as weeds may strangle an untended garden.

In Jordan's case, this was a part of his issue, though not all of it. He certainly had a strained relationship with his mother, and hardly any relationship at all with his father, and there was little doubt that a dark, deeply hidden part of him was drawn toward death as the result of hopelessness.

First and foremost, a patient in such a state must realize that what they are experiencing is not all that life has to offer; indeed, the state of hopelessness is only a sad parody of life. In a sense, a person stuck in such a state is not really living at all; they are experiencing a sort of living death. All ego-bound states create conflict and depression to some degree. It is only when this becomes the dominant state that desperation ensues.

The only way for the patient to recover from this is to endeavor, fully and with as much dedication as they can summon, to learn through direct experience how joy, peace, and hope *can* be found in life. Obviously, this entails some changes; however, this does not mean behavioral shifts are necessary as much as emotional and thought-based ones. The realization of joy is actually an easy one to make once the patient's direction of searching has been adjusted. The shift into joy is indeed a tiny movement. Within each of us, a blazing light exists at the center of our beings, which anyone can touch and which takes only an instant to connect with. Experiencing this can rapidly transform a patient's outlook on life, which is one reason connecting with the healing dimension sparks such profound healing.

Sickness and Body Identification

There is saying about disease: "The *I* in *illness* is isolation, and the crucial letters in *wellness* are *we*." Disease *is* isolation. It involves an explicit cutting off from others, a battening down and tightening up of the physical boundaries that seem to separate us from the world and people around us. It solidifies the sense that we are alone and safely isolated within the framework of the body's walls.

Although I didn't realize it at the time, I now see that this was Jordan's major underlying problem. Curiously, this particular cause of disease is the one most likely to afflict the spiritually evolved. Even though Jordan was only eighteen years old at the time his crisis began, and not at all overtly interested in spirituality, I later recognized that he was an advanced soul.

My hunch that this was true began when I noticed how responsive his body was to his mental state. While everyone's body responds to the mind, the connection is rarely as blatant as it was in Jordan's case. His physical responses to emotional crises, as well as positive states, were rapid and powerful. It was as if there was no buffer whatsoever between his mind and body. Virtually every severe medical setback he endured followed some major blowup with someone he was close to. The connection was hard to miss. So as his chemotherapy treatments failed one by one and winter gave way to spring, the realization that his disease was clearly paralleling his emotional state prompted me to set aside whatever hesitance I felt about teaching Jordan to meditate and begin working with him more directly.

I started by leading him through occasional, simple relaxation exercises. When these went well, I began guiding him through more detailed visualizations that focused on healing imagery (I discuss this more in part 3). As it turned out, Jordan showed no resistance at all to meditation — indeed, just the opposite. To my surprise he genuinely enjoyed the practice, and he took to it far more intuitively than most of my students, including some who had been practicing meditation for years. Eventually Jordan even enrolled in an eight-week meditation class I was teaching at a local hospital, and he enthusiastically attended all but one of the sessions.

When I later interviewed Jordan for this book, he told me that meditation has changed his life forever, and he still practices regularly. He said it's something that he expects will always be a part of his life.

To appreciate why the spiritually advanced are prone to this source of disease, consider the purpose the physical body serves. In Earth School the body is a structure that functions much like a wall. It marks out your "territory," separating your life and existence from everyone else's and shutting out perceived outsiders. Essentially, the boundaries of your body map out, in your own perspective, where you end and the rest of the universe begins, much as a fence around your yard delineates your property line.

Almost nobody in the world views the body in this way. Most people think of the body as what and who they are, not as a fence *surrounding* who and what they are. Yet it remains true that the life within your fence is not the same as the structure that surrounds it, just as the fence around your property is not itself your home. The fence merely marks your personal territory. The spark of life that is within you, located beneath the heavy layers of ego and your physical identification, is what you are, and it is this part of you that is eternal. The life that is within is not actually bound by or restricted to your personal fences in any way, at any time. You can come and go at will as often as you please, just as you freely come and go to and from your physical home. It is only fear that keeps you from doing so.

When we become adapted to living within the confines of the ego and the physical body, we literally become afraid of going beyond them, just as a bird that has been raised in captivity may fear leaving its cage when it is liberated. This is a deep-set, hidden fear all human beings have in common. If you were to relinquish this fear, you would instantly become a visionary. In short, you would see God — *everywhere*. Subconsciously we believe that if we were to go beyond our limited walls, we would be swept away into oblivion by the vastness of inner space. The ego is so terrified of your core Self, it would rather you die than see what lies beyond it.

Put simply, sickness is a way of reinforcing your identification with your fence — your body and ego. Disease, therefore, is really a symptom of the fear of enlightenment. It reaffirms yourself as a separate entity, rather than as a part of everything and everyone in the living universe, which is what enlightenment truly is.

This bodily reinforcement operates through the explicit use of discomfort and pain. When you are sick, or in pain of any sort, your connection to your body is amplified. You therefore feel temporarily safe from the "threat" of drifting outside your physical walls and catching a glimpse of your Self. This is why spiritually advanced souls are so prone to this form of illness. They are very close to the realization that they are more than a body, and that it is indeed quite easy — not to mention pleasurable — to go beyond the physical realm. This causes any sense of ego they still have to become afraid, and in some cases outright desperate.

The answer to this dilemma is to realize that you will not be harmed in any way by exploring inner space and communing with your Self and Source — and then to actually conduct this exploration. Only through confronting the ego's false fears can you learn that they are fully unjustified; in this, only experience can serve as your teacher. All that will happen when you shift into the present and reconnect with your Self is that you will feel immensely peaceful, empowered, and happy. And the deeper your awakening, the more intense these feelings will become.

Awakening is a gentle process, not one that involves force of any kind. It happens only according to your own will, and it proceeds at the pace you alone set. To the extent that you resist it, awakening cannot occur; as you desire it, it happens automatically. Nothing in your life as you know it in Earth School will be attacked or injured in any way during this sacred, healing experience. In practice, the opposite occurs. The body is healed, and negative ego states are gently corrected.

Meditation and related practices are like walking up a quiet garden path that leads from your own backyard into a lush hillside that rises beyond the noise, pollution, and clamor of everyday life. And it is here, from this lifted perspective, that you are able to look back upon what you have left behind from a place of safety and true objectivity. The view from the top affords you a fresh vision, which reveals the world in a whole new light. When you return, you will still have the same house, the same neighbors, and the same job. Only your perspective will have changed.

CHAPTER SEVEN

New Hope: "Smart" Chemo and Bone Marrow Transplants

*I*n our physical world we tend to view ourselves as physical creatures who rely on physical remedies to cure our various physical diseases. As a result, virtually all our faith rests on the shoulders of modern medicine, as opposed to spiritual and emotional therapies. Not surprisingly, this was true in Jordan's case as well. Even from my own perspective, I invested so much faith in the medical system that, when his third round of chemo failed miserably, my hope, along with the hopes of everyone who loved Jordan, was dashed to pieces and scattered by the winds of misplaced faith, leaving me feeling empty and sick with impending doom.

It began to feel as if the harder we attacked Jordan's cancer, the stronger and more aggressive it became. By this time, his treatment options had been exhausted, and even though Dr. Martin went straight to work fishing for other possibilities, none of us were particularly optimistic. By now Dr. Martin had started to broach the subject that in all probability Jordan would need a bone marrow transplant in order to survive. One of the most brutal and dangerous medical procedures being performed today, it is used only as a last resort in order to save a patient's life. Unfortunately, the procedure is so hazardous that Jordan's disease needed to be under control before he would be eligible to receive one. Also, because of the complexity and expense of the treatment, it can take months to set up and find a suitable donor who is deemed a good genetic match for the patient.

Bone Marrow Transplants

Bone marrow transplants are delicate undertakings that can easily prove fatal. There is decidedly little room for error. The aim of the procedure is to replace dysfunctional blood stem cells with healthy ones. Stem cells can be thought of as seeds. While this analogy isn't perfect, it's close enough. Blood stem cells "grow" white blood cells (which fight infection), red blood cells (which carry oxygen), and platelets (which help the blood to clot and prevent bleeding). The goal of a bone marrow transplant is to permanently destroy the patient's current supply of unhealthy blood stem cells and replace them with new, functioning ones, which will be better equipped to fend off disease.

The patient's immune system is completely destroyed during this process; hence the patient's symptoms need to be under control before the transplant can be performed. In Jordan's case, given his weakened condition and the active flaring of his disease, the procedure was deemed too dangerous. He was caught in a classic catch-22: he needed this desperate procedure because he was desperately ill, yet he couldn't receive it until he got better.

Bone marrow transplants work to cure lymphoma in a couple of ways. First of all, the patient is given whopping doses of chemo drugs and, in some cases, is blasted with radiation. This process is intended to obliterate as many cancer cells as possible, but it also simultaneously destroys the patient's bone marrow — the body's manufacturing plant of blood cells and, by extension, the engine of the immune system.

Without healthy bone marrow and a functioning immune system, the body would be quickly overrun by disease-causing organisms and the patient would soon perish. Because of this, during the procedure, patients are isolated from the outside world in a sealed ward that utilizes a positive pressure system to ensure a near-sterile environment.

Positive pressure works by maintaining a greater air pressure within the treatment ward than in the surrounding facilities so that unfiltered airflow into the controlled environment is reduced. When you open the door to enter a positive pressure ward, you are hit by a gentle, steady breeze as air from within rushes outward, thus controlling any possible contamination from outside. Guests are typically only allowed to visit during less-critical phases of the patient's treatment. They are admitted through a monitored security door and must wash their hands for a full minute or more using a medical soap before being allowed inside. They are also strictly screened to ensure they are not ill; visitors must sign a form swearing that they have suffered no symptoms of any infectious disease in recent days, such as from the flu or a cold.

Places like this become a sort of sanctuary for patients with absolutely no functioning immune system to protect them from a world riddled by viruses, bacteria, and parasites. During this highly precarious stage of the treatment, while the body's defenses are down, even the most minor infection can prove fatal.

The patient is then given bone marrow cells from a donor who has been carefully screened and selected for his or her genetic similarity to the patient. These matches are rarely, if ever, perfect — even when the donor is a close relative — and an imperfect match can cause serious side effects after the procedure, such as graft-versus-host disease, which is a condition that causes the new immune system to attack the patient's own body. This reaction occurs when the donated immune system (or graft) fails to recognize the patient's body (the host) as equivalent to itself, and so it does exactly what it is designed to do — *it attacks the invader.* Graft-versus-host disease can lead to chronic problems that can plague the patient for years or, off and on, for the remainder of their life. It can affect the patient's liver, stomach, skin, mucous membranes, lungs, and the immune system itself, causing a host of painful, and in some cases debilitating, symptoms, such as explosive diarrhea, horrible rashes, pneumonia, liver damage, and other unpleasant complications.

Curiously, the tendency of the grafted immune system to attack the host is also the primary way in which bone marrow transplants operate to heal lymphoma. In cases like Jordan's, part of what often happens is that the immune system is no longer identifying cancer cells as dysfunctional, and thus it is not doing a very good job of eliminating them. This allows the cancer to flourish at will and eventually overrun the patient's body. When the new immune system is put into place, it is better able to correctly identify and destroy whatever cancer cells have managed to survive the huge doses of chemo and radiation. If all goes well, the patient emerges on the other end of this process cancer free.

As gruesome as all of this sounds, after the chemotherapy had failed to cure Jordan, a bone marrow transplant appeared to be his best hope. However, we were told that his disease would have to be controlled for perhaps as long as two or three months in order for him to receive the transplant, and this appeared to be an insurmountable hurdle. Although Jordan's medications had gotten more aggressive as his treatments went along, so had his disease. Since he had fallen ill, Jordan hadn't spent more than a few weeks without symptoms, much less months, and things only seemed to be getting worse.

The situation seemed utterly impossible. How could we find a way to halt the cancer's advance and beat it back long enough to find a donor, set up a transplant, and allow Jordan the chance to sufficiently recover? At this dark moment in Jordan's journey, the final conclusion, given all his complications, was that we couldn't even consider a transplant, though there was nothing else to consider.

Or was there?

Targeted Chemotherapy

It was at this point that Dr. Martin hit on a possible solution, "targeted chemotherapy," and this resurrected our hopes yet again. Mind you, we were desperate. We had seen treatment after treatment knocked flat, and we were beginning to expect the worst. When this happens, it only makes a grim situation all the grimmer. Negative expectations have a nasty tendency to increase the possibility of negative outcomes, given the powerful influence of the mind. In this circumstance, with Jordan's situation feeling so precarious, and his suffering so acute, we clung to any little scrap of hope like a shipwreck survivor adrift in the water, grasping at a floating chunk of debris — clinging to anything that might help us hold our heads above water.

All throughout his body, Jordan's lymph nodes had now swollen up to the size of golf balls again. In particular, one was lodged against his liver and causing him severe distress. He was in agony, and there was nothing we could do to help him. To watch someone you care about struggle and suffer so deeply, and to be utterly unable to help, is one of the purest forms of torture I have ever encountered. This psychological agony can cause some family and friends to pull away and separate themselves from the situation in order to shield themselves from the pain.

If you are a close to someone who is ill and you feel a desire to isolate yourself, first of all, *do not feel guilty!* Understand that such reactions are natural, and I suspect virtually everyone who has witnessed a loved one in pain has experienced this to some degree. There may well be times when you *do* need to withdraw from a patient's side in order to clear your mind and gather your strength. Take this time when you need to, and do so with a clear conscience. A loved one's welfare depends, in part, on the emotional stability of his or her caregivers, and if they become mentally exhausted, they will be of little help. So *do* periodically take a break, withdraw, and forget about the situation as best as you are able. Get away. Relax. Try to rest. And do whatever helps to take your mind off the stress. Watch a movie. Treat yourself to a nice dinner. Get a massage. Laugh whenever possible (there is no better medicine than laughter). Get some exercise, whether it involves going on a walk, a hike, or a run, taking a yoga class, or hitting the gym for weight training.

Then, when you are ready, return to your loved one's side. Despite how difficult the situation may be, remember that he or she *needs* you more than you can know. Nobody heals in isolation. Your care helps provide the strength, faith, and drive for the patient to recover. Therefore your presence is a vital, irreplaceable component to the healing process. Above all, do not ever forget this.

In Jordan's case, we were all tired by this point, not to mention thoroughly traumatized, though most of us tried to hide our fear for his sake. Acute fear states are exhausting, like treading water. You can only do it for so long.

When I interviewed Brittany for this book, she said she intentionally tried to treat Jordan the same way she would normally treat him if he wasn't sick. That is, she didn't baby him, except by taking up a ritual in which she would regularly kiss him on the cheek and tell him that each kiss was medicine to help him heal.

It is true that sometimes a patient just needs to be treated like a regular person. For patients one of the most stressful components of a serious disease is watching their loved ones suffer, so it is wise to mitigate this perception to whatever extent possible. It is important — indeed vital — to let them know you care, but it is equally valuable to remain a positive, vital force in their life.

Targeted chemotherapy, which is also sometimes called "smart therapy," is a relatively new form of chemo. In the past it was only available to treat a few forms of cancer, but the number of cancers now being treated by targeted therapy is booming. This type of treatment is an exciting, cutting edge frontier in the world of cancer treatments, born from our massively expanding scientific, technological, and medical knowledge, and it represents the approach medicine will likely be using more frequently in the years to come. Dr. Martin described the difference between standard chemotherapy and targeted therapy as being like the difference between trying to destroy cancer by hitting the patient with a baseball bat versus sending in trained sharpshooters to target the cancer cells directly.

As it turned out, a targeted medication had just become available only months before that was designed to treat Jordan's particular form of lymphoma. The timing of this seemed nothing short of miraculous. If Jordan had fallen ill only a few months earlier, he might not have had this fallback option at this critical moment in his journey.

There are a number of types of targeted therapies. In Jordan's case, antibodies, which were armed with small doses of a chemo drug, were used to directly seek and destroy the cancer cells. Antibodies are natural soldiers that the immune system employs to hunt down foreign invaders and dysfunctional cells in the body, such as cancer. All healthy immune systems make them, and each type of antibody specializes in attacking particular invaders or cells. They are like smart missiles that lock onto exact coordinates: you arm, aim, and launch them, and they find the bad guys and take them out (or, in some cases, they tag sickened cells or invaders with a biological marker so another of the immune system's hunter cells can find and neutralize them).

The result of this therapy is that the cancer cells take the bulk of the damage while the rest of the patient's body remains relatively unaffected. That is, relative to traditional chemotherapy; there are still some nasty side effects. These treatments are hardly perfect. But in practical terms, the patient does not experience the same dangerous dip in immune functioning, nor the severe enervation, that occurs during traditional chemo.

Jordan began the targeted therapy as soon as Dr. Martin could lay his hands on the drug, within a matter of days. At that point, Jordan received weekly intravenous transfusions, essentially pumping his body full of "soldiers" who were specially trained to track and defeat an enemy we ourselves could not see. We only knew of their presence due to the damage they inflicted upon Jordan's failing body. Otherwise this enemy was as silent and invisible as it was deadly. The battle to come would be an equally invisible one, with the battlefield being Jordan's lymph system.

This was also the period when I began supplementing Jordan's treatments with guided meditation that included healing imagery. Sometimes I was able to lead him through healing visualization exercises while he was actively receiving his treatments, during doctor appointments, or immediately afterward in the hopes of helping him to activate the natural healing power of his mind, thus amplifying the physical treatments.

Over the weeks to come, Jordan responded well to this

therapy, and to our meditations, and I for one thought this new form of smart chemo was just the miracle we had been praying for. While most people think of miracles as spontaneous healings with no medical intervention involved, I believe that Source actively works through our physicians, nurses, and medications. Not everyone is in a position or a state of mind to receive direct healing. In fact, it is safe to say that most patients are not, so sometimes Source's help comes to us in the form of a pill or, in this case, an intravenous solution.

Whether miraculous or not, Jordan's energy quickly improved, and his white cell count steadily climbed, indicating that his immune system was getting stronger. His pain all but vanished as his lymph nodes shrunk, appearing virtually normal for a change. His smile returned and his face took on the color of life, replacing the sick pallor we had come to know too well.

Three weeks passed...

Then four...

At the five-week mark, Jordan still seemed to be doing great. This was a notable moment, as Jordan had not felt this well for this long a stretch since the disease had first come crashing into his life.

At last we all began to relax and let our guards down. *Again.*

Okay, Jordan is going to make it after all, I told myself. It seemed this smart therapy had arrived just in time, a Divine intervention, and I intuitively liked this treatment for many reasons. It made sense. It felt *right.*

At this point I began forcefully pushing any negative thoughts I became aware of away and out of my mind, replacing them with affirmations intended to shield me from fear: *The antibodies will do the job they are designed to do and rid Jordan's body of cancer. They are Spirit's warriors. They are experts at their function. Everything is going to be all right.* I repeated these thoughts, silently, like a mantra. I got to the point where, in my mind's eye, I could almost *see* the process occurring.

"Everything is going to be fine," I assured Jordan.

"Jordan is going to make it," I told Brittany privately.

Then, at week six of the treatment, Jordan had a huge fight with a friend of his who had allegedly stolen some money from him. Jordan had been saving up so that when the time came for him to get a bone marrow transplant he would have money to support himself while he was in Portland. Of course, Jordan would be housed in the transplant center during and immediately after the transplant, but he would be required to remain in Portland for several months afterward so he could be closely monitored. Within days after this fight, Jordan began having trouble breathing. This was when the real terror began.

CHAPTER EIGHT

The Patient Must Feel
They Deserve to Heal

S pecial Principle of Healing 2 implies that in order for a patient
to *want* to heal, they must also believe they deserve to heal.
Thus Special Principle 3 might be considered a subset of Special
Principle 2, but it is of such critical importance to our state of
health and happiness that it deserves detailed consideration.

> ## Special Principle of Healing 3
> **The patient must feel they deserve to heal.**

In Special Principle 2, we examined how wanting to heal is a
necessary condition for healing to occur. But consider what happens when people do not see themselves as deserving of health.
When this is the case, how can people *want* to heal if they think
they do not deserve to heal?

. The basic tenet at work in Special Principle 3 has already
been touched on: guilt is anger directed inward, and as such it is
the primary emotional fuel of disease. Guilt literally represents

self-attack on the mental level, from which physical attack, or sickness, is destined to follow. Of all the dark emotions at work in the human psyche, guilt is the most directly destructive. In simplest terms, the guilty cannot accept healing because they do not believe they merit it. It doesn't matter how hard they try to recover, nor how advanced the treatments they receive may be. The most progressive, potent medications available will not cure a guilt-driven illness while the guilt remains intact and unchallenged. This is like claiming to be cured of lymphoma merely because the lymph nodes are no longer swollen. The retreat of symptoms does not necessarily indicate a healed condition.

Nor does it matter if guilt lies hidden and locked away in the depths of unawareness. Guilt cannot be hidden away, denied, or disguised. On the contrary, it must be clearly recognized, released through forgiveness, and healed through the active cultivation of love. Invisible guilt will still produce an equally negative effect on the individual. Just as a person's ignorance about the presence of a physical illness will not make the illness disappear, so too is it with the malady of guilt. When there is a guilty conscience, the patient will become stuck in a destructive sequence called *the guilt cycle*, which is destined to result in various physical and mental ailments until it is interrupted. For many people the guilt cycle is a lifelong affliction. Yet if a patient wishes to recover fully, no matter what the illness happens to be, it is vital to understand how this psycho-physical disorder operates and, most important, how to undo it at its foundation.

The Guilt Cycle

Readers of my previous book *Everyday Meditation* are already familiar with the theory of the guilt cycle. Many spiritual seekers believe that the goal of the curriculum of awakening is to overcome worldly desires. But this objective is not nearly as important as the surmounting of guilt. Defeat guilt, and you conquer fear; defeat fear, and you conquer the world. Perhaps this sounds like an exaggeration, but this is not so. Without fear nothing can hold you back from God realization, for I have realized that fear *is* the veil that seems to shut us out from Spirit. Yet it is only an illusion of a veil, generated and maintained by the thinking, ego mind.

The veil of fear is maintained and continuously reinforced through guilt. Everyone in the world is infected with guilt to some degree. It is the disease of our kind, and it is built into the ego's whole thought system. This is what makes the undoing of guilt so powerful. In the ultimate sense, it represents the undoing of the ego, which is the primary cause of suffering, whatever form it may take. This is not something I am going to try to convince you of. I realize that it may, at first, be difficult to believe that guilt has such an enormous impact on our lives. Some people even maintain that guilt is healthy in the sense that it keeps us from hurting others and committing moral and legal crimes. However, guilt is not nearly as effective at preventing crime as love is. The reason I do not wish to hurt others is not because I would feel guilty if I did, but because it would cut me off from the state of love, gratitude, and appreciation for all life that makes my experience on earth meaningful and joyous.

Even those who remain unaware of the guilt within them still experience its effects: sickness, depression, addiction, self-loathing, and anxiety are all the result of unhealed guilt, as are many other forms of suffering. This is why it is so important for students of awakening and students of health alike to become willing to dig into their own minds in order to uncover any negatively charged emotional debris that may be hidden there, so that it can then be forgiven and released. There is no other way to disrupt the guilt cycle.

A further point that needs illuminating involves guilt's origin.

Most people think guilt comes from "immoral" or dishonest behavior, but such things merely add reinforcement to guilt that is already present. The guilt cycle actually began the moment we were born into the world. It originated within you, and it can be found in everyone who walks the earth. According to *A Course in Miracles*, guilt came into existence simultaneously with the belief in separation from God. We use the word "belief" here only because the separation never actually happened. It is an *appearance*, not a fact, and as such it can be likened to an illusion. In Reality, we are all still united with our Source and with each other. This is something you can learn to experience for yourself, so you do not have to take my word for it.

Yet this illusion spawned the darkest of all human emotions, which acts as the primary fuel for our continued sense of division from the rest of the universe. In this way, guilt was not only born through separation, it actively reinforces and maintains it. This is also why blame, "finger pointing," anger, shame, and attack are such a prominent part of the world we live in.

In the name of healing, let us set aside any fear or discomfort we may feel surrounding this subject and take a closer look at the guilt cycle. First of all, on a theoretical level, the reason the belief in separation arouses such deep-rooted guilt is because it makes us feel as if we have attacked the universe by essentially tearing ourselves away and establishing ourselves as independent entities (egos attached to bodies). While we may not actually be separated from the universe in Reality, the belief that we are is strong, and it seems very real during our lives in Earth School. You literally live in Spirit, which is all-encompassing. Even now you are surrounded by Source and immersed in it, though you may be temporarily unable to perceive it. Your life is entirely dependent on your Source. You could not exist apart from God any more than the wind could exist independently from the air.

Once, years ago, I attended a meditation class at the dharma center in Portland, Oregon. I was there as a student, not in the capacity of a teacher — my usual role — which allowed me the freedom to sit back and soak up the atmosphere of the class. I had never tried the particular form of meditation they advocated, which is a type of mindfulness undertaken while the eyes are kept open. The teacher instructed us to rest our gaze a few feet ahead, trying not to focus on any thing or person in particular. The visual field in general was to serve as the focus of this mindfulness practice, or the "ground" that connected us to the present moment. (To be mindful merely means to be aware. The breath is most commonly used as a central focus during mindfulness, but other sensations can be used.)

At some point during the meditation, I began to notice that the room, the objects in the room, and even the bodies of the other students were taking on a peculiar look. Quite suddenly everything seemed unreal, as if it were nothing more than the set and props of a stage play. Everything in the room looked composed of plaster and cardboard that had been artificially painted over. It was as if none of it was real, but just a bunch of miscellaneous stuff that had been thrown together for the sake of appearances.

Just as I noticed this, I began to see little edges of golden light surrounding the objects and people in my visual field. I quickly realized I was having a mystical experience, and I endeavored to relax even more and allow the unfolding vision to progress. I'd had mystical experiences many times during meditation before, so this was not frightening to me, though I'd never had one of such depth with my eyes open. While I was familiar with the sensation of the mystical experience, I had never really seen what the world looked like during it. What occurred next proved to be an utterly fascinating experience, which I will never forget.

Gradually, as I settled more deeply into this state, the light surrounding everything became increasingly brilliant, while the delineations between the people and objects in the room became fuzzy and less defined. As this occurred, the room simultaneously filled with a blazing, golden light, which even made the air itself sparkle and appear luminescent. This effect increased until it appeared to me that the entire world was made up only of this beautiful glowing effervescence — a vast, interconnected field of energy.

It is interesting to note that physicists have known for decades that the universe is actually composed of nothing but pure energy, which is all identical in nature. We cannot ordinarily see this with our eyes, but it is, nevertheless, the true nature of the material objects that make up the physical universe. Scientists have also come to understand that every cell in existence, no matter its physical location — whether it resides within your own body here on Earth, inside a rock on the surface of Mars, or in a hydrogen firestorm on a distant star at the far end of the cosmos — are all somehow, astonishingly, directly connected with one another. As Nobel Prize–winning physicist Erwin Schrödinger once put it, "Quantum physics thus reveals the basic oneness of the universe." At last science and spirituality agree on something!

The reality is, if we were blessed with eyes that could penetrate the true nature of existence, we would see exactly what I *did* see that day in meditation class: a vast, endless sea of interconnected light, from which all life and objects arise and are made manifest in the world of the physical. The dance of form is but a show of light, and the appearance of our separateness can thus be considered a system of illusion, or perhaps more accurately, *delusion*. The vision I had that day was but a glimpse of the truth behind the smokescreen of our worldly existence, and through it I was afforded a rare and stunning insight into the nature of our Reality — yours, mine, and everyone's, for as it turns out, it is all really the same. It does not matter what religion you are, what your nationality is, the color of your skin, where or when you were born in the world, or what language you happen to speak. The differences that appear to separate us can be no more real than the separation of the wind from the air. We have all been created from the same great Energy System, and it is something we are intimately bound to forever.

You could not be alive if you were not still joined to this Field any more than you could watch television on a set with no power connected to it. It is the elemental Energy behind your mind and thoughts, your body, and every object, whether inanimate or animate, that you see surrounding you. Look up into the sky at night — light and life are *everywhere!* And you live in the midst of it. Life is your home, which you have never been apart from for a single instant of your existence.

The trouble is, the moment we disassociated ourselves from this Field of light and life, guilt was born into our thoughts like a curse of madness. Ever after, each of us has been inwardly longing for Home — the place that we know, in our hearts, must still exist though it seems to be lost; it is *we* who are lost. It has never changed nor shifted nor moved its position. Only guilt caused a wall of fear to rise between our self and our Self.

The undoing of guilt involves a state of dreaming as well, but it is a different version of dreaming. It is a dream of healing the separation and of coming Home. It is a dream of awakening from the sleep of separation.

If you monitor your thoughts and interactions with others carefully and with honesty, you can observe the guilt cycle in action. It works like so: you feel guilty, and with that guilt comes the urge to get rid of it. It does not matter *how* you free yourself from it, so you begin searching the world for things, events, and people that displease you and seem, in your own judgment, to be more guilt-ridden than you feel you are. This is not a conscious process. It merely is something we do as if responding to a program. It goes on all the time in virtually everyone. During the process, anyone or anything will do, so long as you can find a way to project your own sense of guilt onto them and away from you. This is the primary impetus for attack and hatred.

As already noted, this system of alleviating guilt through assault never actually works. If it did, there would be no problem because we would all have freed ourselves from guilt long ago, which clearly has not happened. In fact, anger and attack merely reinforce the guilt we already feel. This is precisely the problem with the world and why it seems incapable of any form of lasting healing, peace, and happiness. The only solution to this problem is to undertake a systematic healing approach that seeks to disrupt the guilt cycle and thus liberate us from its vicious, circular toxin. Let's recap:

- Guilt leads to anger, and anger reinforces guilt, which then creates an urge to project guilt again and again and again. As it does, your sense of guilt will cause you to subconsciously sabotage your life and relationships, and punish yourself in one form or another, whether through disease or depression or fear. While guilt remains in your mind, you will endlessly feel depressed, anxious, empty, and angry, though you will not understand why.
- This cycle will not end until you consciously interrupt it.
- Forgiveness of others, self-forgiveness for your own mistakes, the development of compassion and kindness for all living creatures, and the cultivation of unconditional love is the way to break the guilt cycle. You must become actively

committed to exchanging all your negative impulses to attack and blame for characteristics that realign you with Source and your Self, thus ending your sense of separation.

Breaking the Guilt Cycle

Life is simple. Therefore, healing is also simple. It doesn't require complex treatments, medications, or therapies, though these are apt to be a part of most patients' healing regimen, if nothing else simply because people believe in them. The ego is a system of thought rooted in, and thus forever bound to, complexity. Convolution is a key ingredient in the ego's defensive network, which seeks to protect itself by making what is very simple appear to be too complicated to see through and thus escape. Look upon the world, the home of egos and bodies, and you will see endless variations, shades of color, types of life, and shapes, sizes, weights, and heights, as well as an endless list of diseases and their respective "remedies." As we have said, none of these differences actually exist, not in Reality, but it does not matter whether you believe this assertion or not. Healing does not even require that much of you. Once again, only the very simple is asked.

Differences create complexity, and what is complex and divided becomes vulnerable by its very nature. This is clear even within simple worldly terms. Mechanical engineers know this to be true. For instance, the more parts that go into a machine's design, the more likely something will break or go wrong. Another good example of this in physical terms is that a whole, unbroken beam is stronger than one that has been cut and attached back together by bolts.

Healing requires you to take a step back from all the complexity of the world, the variances of form, the differences and the divisions, the opinions of this doctor versus that doctor, the medications and their side effects, and focus on some basic healing principles instead. Forget about how difficult healing seems to be according to the world's dictates; the world knows little of healing, for it does not even know where, and how, life originated, which is the same Source healing derives from. How could it understand healing when it does not understand the cause of life?

The end of guilt is the end of sickness. Like all things about awakening, releasing guilt is a simple process. This is so because guilt always requires you to focus on the past, and the past *is* gone. It no longer exists at all, except in the mind of those who actively choose to focus on it, and by doing so force the past to remain with them. Ending guilt asks only that you accept what is right now, and stop forcing your mind to dredge up and continually relive old wounds, pains, and regrets. Forget the past; it is gone and is therefore unreal. Healing can only occur by aligning with Reality, which is located in the present.

Consider how focusing on the past also reinforces our false sense of separation. The past usually emphasizes those things that set you apart from others — grievances, superiority, inferiority, guilt, and so on, thus making you feel different, either for the better or the worse, it does not matter which.

Many spiritual seekers view time as an enemy, but this is not so. Viewed correctly, time is actually a healing device. The temporal flow is like a river that continuously flows through you. In each instant of its passage you are born again and cleansed of all your past actions and mistakes. Time sweeps them clean and liberates you from their ill effects, carrying away all your pain, guilt, and errors into oblivion and purifying you with every fresh instant. No effort on your part is required for this to happen. It goes on all the time, every moment, whether or not you are aware of it. It is only your own clinging to old thoughts, dead ideas, and painful errors that keeps your past alive and real for you. Karma is but a belief fostered by the ego that you can never be free of the past, or that your release must be postponed until a magical future point arrives that is as equally imaginary as the past itself is. As with the past, there is no future! Only the present is real, or ever will be real.

Do not cling to the past, nor the future, but come to understand the passage of time for what it really is — a liberating force, not a prison house, from which you need no release, for the *now* is eternal and always present. So too is it with the body. You have no need to be freed from either one, nor the karma that so many believe binds them to lifetimes of meditation and service in order to be undone. Your past and your karma *are gone*. You are limited and held prisoner only by the bars of your own belief. Time cannot keep you from immediate liberation, unless you would keep yourself limited and held prisoner.

Guilt is the weapon the ego uses to hold you prisoner to the past. Free yourself from guilt and present healing will no longer be feared. Here is a series of simple steps to get you started:

Stop Reinforcing the Guilt

As a part of his prescribed Eightfold Path, the Buddha instructed his followers, "Guard your thoughts, words, and deeds." This is how many disciples begin their first, uncertain steps toward enlightenment, and to be successful advancing along your path, this must eventually become a daily focus; at first, it needs to be intentionally practiced, and then, as its benefits are realized, it becomes a way of life. You may begin this process at the behavioral level, by "guarding" what you say and what you do, although this step eventually should saturate your thoughts as well because internalized anger has the same effect as externally expressed anger. So you will have to find a way to break this cycle at a much deeper level than by merely changing your behavior alone.

It is also true that the depth of the animosity you harbor does not matter. A little annoyance has the same capacity to destroy your peace as does rage because true peace is a total state. If its opposite is present at all, peace vanishes from your mind entirely. Both anger and peace cannot be found in the same place at the same moment, any more than cold and hot can coexist.

Change Your "Self-image"

This next step is a gentle one that may sound superfluous. If the goal of awakening is to transcend the little, personal self entirely, what good does shifting one's self-image do? The purpose of this step is really one of transition. Its function is to make the journey easier and more gentle by gradually reducing fear along the way. It does not ask you to abandon your sense of ego altogether, which can, and often does, increase resistance and fear. It only asks that you allow the image you hold of yourself to progressively change from a negative-based perception to one grounded in gentleness.

You, like most people, will probably experience many small shifts in self-image during this extended process, in which you will deviate back and forth between the old and new you, but each shift will bring you closer to an ideal self-image, which, while it may not be your true Self, is close enough to allow an easy transition to that which is real in you. For a time, which may be longer for some than others, these variable visions of yourself may cause you to feel that you have no stable self at all, but this is not the case. Remember, the underlying Self is the part of you that never changes and is therefore always stable. All other states are merely images added onto the Self; that is why they appear to be so unstable. Even before the process of awakening becomes a conscious one, nobody actually holds a stable vision of self. Like clouds, images have no true stability at all, so they are bound to continuously shift with passing circumstances and time. It isn't until your self-image at last merges with your Self that you will grasp what true stability means.

How long this process takes is more in your own hands than you may realize. The sooner you accept a version of yourself that in no way conflicts with the gentleness and unconditional love inherent in your Self, with no exceptions, the sooner your conflict will be over. More and more, everything you do and think must come to reflect your highest Self. You are a natural-born creator, a cocreator of the universe, a Divine spirit in a Divine universe of love and eternal life. If you think of yourself in any other way, you are attacking your true Identity and setting yourself at odds with it. Likewise, to view anyone else in any other light is to separate yourself from them and reinforce your sense of isolation from the universe.

I suggest that each day you meditate on the following mantra until it becomes something you have accepted as a fact:

> I am a divine spirit; a wholly loving, creative, innocent child of a wholly loving, creative, innocent Source. I cannot be apart, nor different, in any way from that which created me. Therefore I am a divine spark of God, which means I cannot be sick, I cannot be separate, and I cannot be made to suffer against my will.

If you told yourself this mantra a thousand times a day, in varying forms, it would not be too much. Ideally, all your thoughts should reflect this sentiment because it is the truth and thus realigns you with that which has always been true within you, though it may have been buried under layers upon layers of ego. As you release these false self-concepts, you peel back the illusions of the self to eventually discover the Self that thrives at the core of them all — the original blueprint from which your life, as you know it, developed.

Cultivate True Forgiveness, Compassion, and Unconditional Love

This is the direction the new self-image must take, and as you have noticed, it is a major focus of this book. The reason is probably obvious to you by now: love and its cousins, forgiveness and compassion, take us in the opposite direction of the ego, and therefore they open us to healing and to peace. These practices are like stepping stones that carry us safely through the turmoil of guilt and into its relinquishment. With each loving thought you hold, and with each kind gesture you make, a little light is added to the darkness of the ego's domain, shedding its beneficence unto a world desperately in need of illumination and peace.

So much can be said of this holy trinity — forgiveness, compassion, and love — that it is hard to know where to begin. Perhaps the most important point to keep in mind is that each one has true and false versions, which are apt to be confused, but which lead in fundamentally opposite directions. For instance, false forgiveness always feels like a sacrifice. That is, it seems like you are giving up your right to be angry at someone for something they did, but you are getting nothing in return for your gift. When you undertake false forgiveness, you will still be angry and you will still suffer as a result. This is because you have failed to absolve the guilt attached to your grievance, and guilt *is* torture. On the other hand, true forgiveness cannot feel like a sacrifice because it unfailingly brings joy and a sense of fulfillment with it. You can always tell true forgiveness from its artificial counterpart by the transcendent peace that accompanies it.

Similar feelings can be intuited in reaction to false versus true love and compassion. A general rule of thumb is that whatever releases guilt, brings happiness, and heals is authentic, while that which curses, elicits emptiness, and causes sorrow must be false. Telling them apart is simple because they generate starkly opposite responses in the emotional body. You only need examine your own feelings to determine which you have offered.

Accept That Your Core Self Is Already Perfect and Pure

That the core Self is already perfect and pure underlies the first three of our suggestions. Yet like Special Principle 3 itself, which is related to but distinct from the other Special Principles, it is of such importance that it deserves individual attention. The idea is that, in the ultimate sense, breaking the guilt cycle does not involve *doing* anything; it only requires simple acceptance.

Earlier I suggested that time is not an enemy of enlightenment, but rather a purifying force; however, this statement is not completely accurate. The concept is merely a way of giving the student, or patient, a way of reinterpreting time so as to realize that it is not an obstacle to the path to purity, but a help. Yet looking more deeply, time actually does nothing at all, neither good nor bad. It is a mental construct, not a fact at all. As such it is actually neutral, like money. Only your intention assigns it to one category or another, good or evil.

On the one hand, time can be understood as an agreed-upon system for organizing illusory events in space. This is why space and time appear to be connected. It seems like without time everything in space would happen all at once. Yet the temporal projection is primarily a system human beings use to avoid recognizing the now and thereby to remain oblivious to the Self.

Let me explain. The ego continuously draws your attention to the past and future so as to distract you from abandoning it and engaging fully with the present moment, which may rightly be considered the gateway to eternity and Source. On a side note, eternity does not mean *endless* time. Many people suffer this confusion, and as a result think that eternity must therefore be "boring." However, boredom is actually a product of the passage of time itself, and it derives exclusively from the process of removing your awareness from the present and projecting into the future, which is a maneuver rooted in the belief that the present must somehow be unsatisfying. Yet no evaluation could be faultier! Actually, this distortion of what the here and now offers is so twisted, it could only result from a perspective that has already removed itself from all conscious contact with the now. When you engage with the present, you enter a state of being that, on earth, most closely resembles Nirvana. This is why the ego uses time as a defensive mechanism to keep you from engaging with the now. It wants you to spend all your time dwelling on the past or projecting into the future. It does not matter which. Either one will suit the ego's needs just fine so long as you avoid what is here and what is now.

It should be noted that the past and future are also equally useless to you in terms of producing joy. In reality, they explicitly rob you of the possibility of joy by disconnecting you from the only state in which you will ever experience lasting happiness. The now is also the only state in which you will experience reality because only the present *is* real. Everything else must be a mental projection, which is a form of fantasy. This is why only the acceptance of what is now is needed to free you from guilt and thus awaken. The reason for this is simply that there is no guilt in the present, nor any guilt in you, because guilt must always involve a focus on past mistakes — a past that, as we have already emphasized, is not real beyond your own imagining. Therefore you have actually done *nothing* that needs healing, no mistakes you need to make amends for. Another way of saying this is, you do not have to make yourself perfect, or pure, or healed, or holy for God's sake; you *are* holy, and healed, and pure, and perfect already, for God created you that way. You need do nothing at all but connect with that which you are at your center, your *core Self,* which lies beyond all the false images either you, or others, hold of you.

To reiterate, what you are in truth has never changed. It cannot be made to be impure, either through your own actions or anyone else's. Opinions do not influence it; time does not decay it; disease has no impact upon it; it cannot be made homeless or ill, or assaulted in any way, in any form. When you identify with this part of your Self, you are made immediately safe, instantly at home.

Nothing you have ever done has changed this Divine Self. Thus there is nothing you need to be forgiven for. When you sleep at night, you dream, but in the morning when you awaken, you know that the things that happened in your dream never really occurred, and so your actions were irrelevant to what, and who, you truly are. Dreams have no power to either imprison or liberate. They are fantasies. When you discover the Real in you, you will understand that the same is true of your life in Earth School. Time is not your prison any more than your body is. The cage door has never been locked. You are free.

PART THREE

Methods of Healing

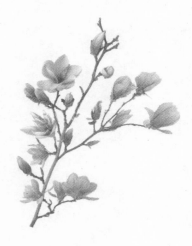

Who is the physician? Only the mind of the patient himself. . . .
Special agents seem to be ministering to him, yet they but give
form to his own choice. He chooses them in order to bring tangible
form to his desires. And it is this they do, and nothing else.
They are not actually needed at all. The patient could merely
rise up without their aid and say, "I have no use for this."
There is no form of sickness that would not be cured at once.

— *A COURSE IN MIRACLES*

CHAPTER NINE

Reprogramming
the Waterfall of Thought

*I*n one sense the methods of spiritual healing all resemble those of physical treatments. That is to say, they are specific techniques you employ in order to stimulate healing. Strictly speaking, though, healing is not dependent on them any more than on medical interventions. As the passage from *A Course in Miracles* that opens part 3 suggests, such remedies, whether physical or metaphysical, merely "give form to" the patient's "own choice," meaning the patient's wish to heal. In other words, such treatments make the healing process *tangible*. For students of Earth School who are thoroughly entrenched in a world based on form, the need for concrete healing agents can be important, even vital in some cases, in order for healing to occur. The crux of the matter is that if you believe such treatments are necessary in order to recover, they probably are. Not as a matter of fact, but strictly due to your own belief in them.

On the other hand, spiritual healing methods are also different than physical treatments in a most profound way in that they are designed to lead you away from the physical and into direct contact with the healing dimension. In this sense they aim to transcend the body and the physical realm entirely, and by doing so provide a much deeper healing experience than any physical remedy could ever hope to accomplish.

Some of the methods presented in part 3 will likely appeal to you more than others, but determining which is most effective for any particular case can be tricky. Actually, people tend to encounter the strongest resistance to those techniques that are most effective. Therefore, I suggest you try all the suggested techniques. Don't dismiss any opportunity to experiment with these valuable exercises, whether you are sick or well. In truth, the ultimate aim and benefit of these techniques has nothing to do with physical healing, which is just a *side effect* of their practice. These are spiritual exercises that, when performed with genuine desire and an open mind, will lead you into direct communion with your Self.

The Waterfall of Thought

Having already introduced the notion of the waterfall of thought, let's examine it and its reprogramming more deeply. Wisdom dictates that all journeys begin in precisely the same place — right *where* you happen to find yourself at the journey's outset, and right *when* you happen to find yourself there. For most of us this means at the level of the body and ego, for this is where our identification is initially centered. Though our goal will lead us inward and far beyond these false images of our self, yet must we begin at the beginning. We cannot do otherwise.

I will leave the physical remedies of disease to the world's physicians, for that is their expertise. My own contribution to healing involves training at the level of thought. It is perhaps one of the most curious things about human nature that the majority of people understand little, if anything, about the nature and power of their own thoughts. Your mind is anything but idle, limited, and weak. Indeed, just the opposite is true. It is an incredibly active force that colors, describes, and influences everything you see and experience each day, all day long, in untold and incalculable ways. There is nothing in your world that is not impacted by your thoughts. Furthermore, as we've noted, it has been estimated that the human mind processes an average of about sixty thousand thoughts per day, which equates to roughly twenty-two million thoughts a year.

Every year.

Consider for a moment the sheer volume of this process: twenty-two million thoughts race through your mind annually; they have done so since you were a young child, and they will continue to do so for the remainder of your life. Over an average lifetime this equates to *billions* of thoughts. For just this reason the thinking process has been compared to "the waterfall of thought," for the stream of inner dialogue is so steady that it is hardly even noticed by many of us, becoming a sort of *white static* in the background of our existence. Our thoughts ramble on and on through our heads in an unbroken stream of run-on sentences, with virtually no pause and precious little conscious intention to guide and evaluate their worth and validity.

Another curious human tendency is to assume that the thoughts passing through our minds are true. I once watched a program on Oregon Public Broadcasting that discussed research identifying the characteristics and habits of the happiest people. A few of these characteristics were obvious, such as that people who forgive others and don't live in the past tend to be happier than those of us who judge and dwell on grievances. Also, people who meditate regularly tend to be some of the happiest people on the planet, regardless of nationality or any other stratifying characteristic. However, one of the traits of happy people caught me off guard. These researchers found that those who do not automatically assume that their thoughts are *true* are happier and better adjusted than others.

What a fascinating discovery! To be honest, I had never even considered that people assume their thoughts to be true, but we do. Most of us identify so closely with our inner dialogue that we believe, without any hesitation or even the slightest questioning, that all these random tidbits of perception racing through our mind are absolutely factual and represent reality.

This is a thoroughly limiting, misleading, and at times dangerous assumption to make. Thinking is a highly personal process, which is based on much more than just what our senses feed to us. The thinking process is tied into an astonishingly complex web of past associations, future anticipations, biases, opinions, likes, dislikes, fears, hopes, dreams, and millions of other considerations that are as unique to you as the constellations that populate the evening sky. Thinking is a system of personal judgment, not fact-sorting.

To add to the confusion, when we are engaged with the ego, our thoughts and body represent our entire universe. The ego knows nothing of the state of being that exists independent of thought, and in fact cannot even conceive of such a state. The ego is literally a prison *built* of thoughts, ideas, and perceptions, which is why egos take their personal beliefs and values with utmost seriousness. When you engage with the ego, you will in essence believe that *you are your thoughts*. This explains the reason many of us become so easily threatened when someone doesn't happen to share our point of view about something. It feels as if they are assaulting a part of what and who we are on a fundamental level by their refusal to share the things we hold to be valuable and true. Yet our thoughts are just images and beliefs we have added onto what we truly are. As such, *none* of them are true. When we are identifying with them, we are therefore equating ourselves with a fantasy, and we are thus dissociating our own reality.

Another obvious problem with identifying too closely with our thoughts is that an extreme number of them are negative in nature, being composed of various judgments, grievances, guilt, anger, feelings of unworthiness, fear, and similarly depressing content. If you identify with these types of thoughts, you are bound to feel depressed, anxious, worthless, and guilt-ridden. You have probably heard the saying, "You are what you eat," and in a physical sense this statement is true enough. The food you consume is broken down by your body and is used as fuel to pro-duce, and sustain, the body's cells. However, it is also true that *you are what you think*. In essence, the thoughts you think make up your mental body. When you identify with your thoughts, you literally *become* what you think. If you fill your mind with fear thoughts, you will become a fearful person, and if you fill your mind with anger and judgment, you will believe yourself to be a judgmental and angry person. Can you really love and respect yourself with such an ugly mental perception?

The unavoidable truth is that unpleasant thinking produces an unpleasant state of mind. At the rate of twenty-two million thoughts per year, how could it not? The happy news is, pleasant thinking creates experiences and emotions in its own likeness as well.

Think of it this way: your inner voice is your constant life companion, the most intimate roommate you will ever have. Imagine if you had a room for rent in your home, and two people came over to view it. Now imagine that the first person turned out to be someone you clicked with right away. She was intelli-gent and friendly, and she had great references and a good job to top it all off. But the second person was a different story alto-gether. Before you even opened the door, you overheard her on the phone yelling at someone. Then, as she toured your place, she complained about everything — the state of your home, the room, the rent, and so on.

Which potential renter would you pick, knowing full well you are going to have to deal with this individual daily?

What you may not realize is you *do* have a renter in your home. This renter is with you always, every second, and there is no way to escape this person because they live inside your own mind. This renter is both your companion — whether friend or foe — and a tour guide who describes everything you see, hear, feel, smell, experience, touch, and taste, and everyone you meet and how you should feel about those relationships, past and present, along with your hopes and fears, dreams and regrets, judgments, what you like, and what you do not like, and every conceivable subject under the sun and stars. This roommate also tells you what you are worth, whether you are a good or bad person, what your value is to the world, what you are capable of accomplishing, and what is beyond your reach because of your limitations, lack of talent, need for more education, losing personality, bad luck, deficient abilities, and on and on...

This force, this mammoth waterfall of thought, may not be what you really are in truth, but while you do identify with it, its impact can hardly be considered inconsequential. On the contrary, your thoughts are one of the mightiest forces that shape your life, just as certainly as a real waterfall alters the terrain it flows through without fail. The millions of words flooding your mind each year describe your *entire* human universe.

And yet, incredibly, we are never taught how important our thinking process is, how it shapes us and affects us. You too may be like so many people who have never given much "thought" to your thoughts. If so, it is time to begin.

Reprogramming the Waterfall

While it is possible to release your identification with the waterfall and temporarily transcend it, doing so is made far gentler through reprogramming its content, during which negative patterns of inner dialogue are healed and transformed into positive talk that does not reinforce guilt and fear. Practically speaking, you cannot *stop* the waterfall any more than you can stop a real waterfall, at least not for long. But you can change its content.

This section could alternately be titled, "Kicking Out Your Wicked Roommate and Inviting In a Friendly One." The first thing to keep in mind is you don't want to fight or argue with the force inside your head. Doing so only fuels conflict, which is what you are attempting to free yourself from. Therefore, this three-step process of transformation is composed of short, gentle practices during which you intentionally identify and replace negative thought habits with positive ones.

1. Bring Awareness to the Waterfall

Begin the reprogramming process by making a regular examination of your thoughts to determine their content. You've already practiced this step earlier in the book. Simply sit down for a few minutes several times a day and let your thoughts run their course, paying attention to their content and general message. What is your roommate saying to you? What is dominating your consciousness? Is it positive or negative in basic scope? Also identify what feelings those thoughts provoke in your perception. If they create anxiety, guilt, fear, anger, or related emotions, they are negatively charged and contribute to unhappiness and disease; on the other hand, if they cause you to feel happy, peaceful, safe, connected to other people, and loved, they are positively charged and contribute to healing. Even the simple process of becoming aware of your thoughts and their effects brings consciousness to the waterfall and will initiate the transformation process.

2. Kick Out Your Wicked Roommate and Invite In a Friendly One

Once you have become familiar with the overall pattern of your thinking process, step two involves challenging any negative thought patterns while encouraging positive ones — but without feeling guilty about having harbored the harmful ones in the first place. It makes no sense to feel guilty when guilt itself is just another negative emotion. The entire purpose of this exercise is to free yourself from such tendencies.

For example, if you want to apply for a new job, you might catch your inner dialogue telling you that you are not qualified, smart enough, or talented enough to get the job. When you recognize this sort of negative self-talk, stop, identify the thought as a negatively charged form of energy, and challenge it by declaring the reverse. Instead, tell yourself, specifically and clearly, that you are qualified, smart enough, and talented enough to land the position.

You get the idea.

At first, focus on challenging the most obvious, dominant negative thoughts that cross your mind. Don't feel that you have to do this with every negative thought that occurs to you. Over time, with practice, a general set will develop, and you will find yourself naturally working through this process without any effort at all.

3. Saturate Your Consciousness with Peace Thoughts

"Peace thoughts" are just what they sound like: words or sentences that are peaceful, empowering, and inspiring. They focus on the beauty of life, joy, connectedness to other people, forgiveness, compassion, cooperation, faith, hope, love, and so on. Start collecting peace thoughts to use in this way. You can find them in many sources, and when you start seeking them, they may suddenly seem to be everywhere. Look for peace thoughts in books, poems, magazines, TV shows, movies, music, and on the Internet. You will also discover many already in your own head amid the flow of thoughts that exist in your personal waterfall.

I suggest you use only one peace thought a day. I have included some examples of ones I have used below, but virtually any inspiring word, sentence, or short paragraph will work. Even single words like "joy," "peace," "calm," or "light" are suitable. Begin first thing in the morning or as soon as possible after waking up. Close your eyes and repeat the peace thought slowly to yourself several times, allowing it and its meaning to saturate your consciousness. Focus all your attention on it and feel as if you are sinking down through your thoughts and toward your core. You may find that this happens quite naturally during this practice. You don't have to *try* to make anything in particular occur. Just focus on letting go, feeling safe, and relaxing.

Practice in this way for at least a few minutes, or continue longer if you enjoy the sense of restfulness it brings. Then, as you go about your day, attempt to recall the peace thought at least once or twice an hour. This only takes a few seconds, so it won't interrupt your normal activities. It is particularly important to call the thought to mind when you experience turbulent emotions, whatever the cause of the upset. Think the peace thought slowly and repeatedly until the negative feeling dissipates.

If you have time, it is helpful during the middle of the day to sit down, close your eyes, and repeat the morning exercise. This will aid you in keeping your thoughts quiet and aligning with the healing space of the now. Even if you are not able to do an afternoon session, you should always close your eyes in the evening and practice with your chosen peace thought before bed. It is important to clear your mind of as many negatively charged emotions as possible before sleeping. This will orient your thoughts toward peace and quietness, and you will benefit from a more restful sleep as a result.

Here are a few examples of peace thoughts to get you started:

- My mind is bathed in quiet stillness; my heart is beating in eternal peace. My body is surrounded by perfect safety; my soul resonates with the joy of Great Spirit.
- In gratitude I choose to spend this day, at one with the present, aware of every passing breath, and awake in the now.
- With each day, and with every newborn instant, am I born again. Now I am free, for the past is gone, and the future is yet to be. I release both, and know myself as I have always been.
- Forgiveness is the path I walk; gentleness is all I see and all I am. Kindness is the gift I give to everyone I look upon and to those who look upon me.
- My body is a holy temple. It is not who I am, but a sacred vessel as I journey through Earth School. I will use it kindly, treat it wisely, and care for it daily. My body is a holy temple. God abides here with me.
- I rest in Spirit. I am Spirit. Spirit is eternal. Spirit is me.
- I am safe. I am healed. I am whole. I am Home.
- Forgiveness, compassion, freedom, release.
- Strength, courage, love.
- Peace, calm, still.
- Joy, light, unity.

CHAPTER TEN

On a Wing and a Prayer

On June 10, 2012, at 10 a.m., I attended the Sunday morning service at the local Unity Center in my area. I am not a regular attendee. As both a writer and a long-term practitioner of meditation, I freely admit to being a bit of a hermit. I enjoy spending most Sunday mornings meditating and studying various spiritual teachings in private. You could say that it is my form of communion with God.

When I do feel compelled to convene with my fellow spiritual journeyers, I often choose Unity. I have found that their message of love, forgiveness, and the acceptance of *all* religious gospels to be uniquely in line with my own beliefs. As it turned out, on this particular morning I was in for a pleasant surprise. A guest speaker had been scheduled, and I found his talk particularly engaging. He was funny, wise, inspiring, and exuded the authentic aura of grounded spirituality that marks all true teachers. I clicked with him immediately, and I was thankful I had decided to abandon my "cave" for a change that morning.

During his presentation I found myself easily transported

beyond my physical environment and into the spiritual realm, and I realized even then, as I sat listening and meditating, that it was no coincidence I had decided to be there that day. "God does not play dice," Albert Einstein once observed, a sentiment I wholeheartedly concur with. Somehow this morning did not feel like a dice game to me. It felt *planned*. So while I listened to the talk, I decided that I was going to introduce myself to this teacher after the service was over, thinking that perhaps we had been meant to meet. However, as it turned out, this was not to be. Instead, this man's visit, along with my communion with my friends and the regular minister of the center, Jane Meyers, was indeed no coincidence — but not for the reason I initially assumed. Only later did I realize the gathering of connected, spiritually grounded souls that morning was actually meant to provide me with the raw spiritual energy I would need during the trial that was to come, which would mark one of the most difficult periods of my life.

I have started to learn that this is precisely how Spirit operates. We often *think* we know what's best for us, and it is inevitable that we try to plan for our future needs based on our own blind anticipations. Yet the truth is that none of us can know a thing about what the future holds for us or anyone else, and therefore we cannot know what we will need in the future, nor what is "best." We are indeed much like little children in this regard. When you align with Source, you gradually come to discover that you no longer have to worry about your future needs. I have found consistently since becoming a conscious student of spiritual awakening that *everything* I have truly required for my journey has somehow manifested itself at just the right moment.

Now, this is not to imply that no planning or action will ever be required on your part from time to time, but even this you do not need to concern yourself with. Whatever guidance you require to plan for the future will also be provided for you in a similarly mysterious fashion. As your trust increases, you will gradually discover that your focus need only remain centered on being quiet enough to hear Source's guidance in the present and on releasing your need to control the events and circumstances of your life.

So, as is typical, that Sunday morning at Unity I made some assumptions about why I was there and planned to introduce myself to the guest speaker after services were over.

But it didn't happen that way...

I do not typically pay attention to my cell phone during spiritual gatherings, and as usual I had my ringer on silent that morning. For some reason, about halfway through the talk, I slipped my phone out of my pocket and noticed that I had received a text. It was from Brittany, and the message instantly set my heart hammering —

"Jordan can't breathe! We're rushing him to the ER!"

I knew Jordan had been experiencing some increased symptoms recently despite the fact that the targeted therapy had been going generally well, but the urgency of Brittany's message caught me totally off guard. I replied that I would meet them at the hospital and hurried for the door. During the short drive, a sense of numbness descended upon me. Even then, long before the doctors confirmed what was happening, something inside me already seemed to know.

The emergency room at St. Charles Hospital immediately took Jordan in and measured his blood oxygen level. It was in the low seventies. The normal level should be in the nineties, and ideally close to one hundred. This indicated a serious problem. Jordan wasn't getting nearly enough oxygen.

The emergency room didn't keep him long. They rapidly, and quite correctly, identified his condition as being serious, and he was transferred to the custody of the hospital's intensive-care unit.

This is where he was when I arrived. Both of my daughters were also there, along with my ex-wife (Brittany's mother), with whom I am still close friends; one of Jordan's friends; and eventually my girlfriend, Kirsten, who would become my wife two years later. We packed the waiting room, trying not to pace the floors, and waited on news. After what seemed like hours, but was really no longer than fifteen or twenty minutes, we were told that one of us could go back to see Jordan and speak with the doctor, and I was nominated.

A nurse led me to a small curtained room where I found Jordan lying on a bed with oxygen tubes feeding into his nose and an IV line infusing him with fluids. It hadn't been long since I had last seen him, but suddenly he looked weaker and more frail than ever, and his face was fully drained of color, lending him a bleached pallor that resembled the white sheet pulled across his abdomen.

I sat at his bedside and the doctor in charge of the ICU joined us within a few minutes. He did not have good news. While they were going to run a test for pneumonia, the doctor didn't seem to think this was the reason for Jordan's difficulty breathing. He implied, though did not say directly, that he thought the cancer had spread into Jordan's lungs. He also suggested that based on Jordan's recent medical history, and the fact that every treatment he had received so far had failed, Jordan's situation was very serious. He told us that Jordan needed to be transported as soon as possible to the hospital at Oregon Health & Sciences University (OHSU) in Portland, which is a level-one trauma center, offering the most progressive treatment available in the state and some of the best in the country. By comparison, St. Charles is a level-two trauma center, which means they can handle just about any emergency. I later learned that St. Charles rarely needs to transfer any of their patients.

The doctor, though he had never met Jordan, seemed to be genuinely intrigued by Jordan's case. By the time we talked, he had already breezed through all of Jordan's medical history, and he wanted to know more about his situation. He asked Jordan a series of questions that seemed primarily designed to satisfy the doctor's curiosity, which Jordan answered patiently. This was the first time that I realized how unusual it was for a person Jordan's age to be diagnosed with this particular form of lymphoma. Most kids get Hodgkin's disease, an infinitely more treatable version of the illness.

In lieu of being able to suggest a treatment plan or provide us with even a hint of hope, the doctor suggested that we consider contacting St. Jude Children's Research Hospital — perhaps the most well known and advanced hospital and research center for youths in the nation — in the hopes they might be able to take Jordan as a patient, or at least offer some possible course of treatment. Clearly, this was a drastic suggestion, since St. Jude is halfway across the country in Memphis, Tennessee, not to mention the fact that Jordan had turned eighteen several months before — a point the doctor himself noted. To me this indicated the seriousness of the situation in a way the medical staff was not ready to openly admit just yet.

The doctor explained to us that they had a difficult decision to make. He felt that Jordan needed advanced care *immediately*, but there was no clear course of treatment available. Therefore St. Charles couldn't do anything for Jordan other than prevent him from presently dying from asphyxiation. Furthermore, they were concerned that if they tried to transport Jordan to OHSU immediately, he might go into respiratory arrest and die on the way.

The decision wasn't settled until later that afternoon. After consulting with OHSU, St. Charles decided to keep Jordan overnight in an attempt to stabilize him, and then a medical transport plane would fly him 175 miles across the Cascade Mountain Range to Portland the next morning.

It was a terrifying choice either way. On the one hand, he was precariously perched on a razor-thin edge between life and death, from which he could easily topple during the short, one-hour flight to Portland. On the other, every moment counted. Jordan was now, quite suddenly, actively, and presently, dying. All we could do was pray that the doctors at OHSU would somehow come up with a miracle solution.

That night, I hardly slept. In the morning, still groggy and in a state of shock, I arranged to take an emergency leave from work. I then e-mailed Jane Meyers, the minister at Unity, and explained Jordan's urgent need. She promised to spread the word and lead Unity's members in focused prayers on his behalf. I know many others were praying for him as well. Whether or not you are a believer in the efficacy of prayer, the psychological support it provides alone is worth the effort.

About the same time Jordan was being loaded onto the airplane that would carry him to OHSU, I hurriedly stuffed a few changes of clothing and some other essentials into a duffel bag, along with a battered copy of *A Course in Miracles*, and tossed the pack into the trunk of my car. I had learned, just that morning, that Jordan's family would not be able to make the trip. A variety of reasons were given for this, but the truth was that it was an emotionally crushing moment for everyone, and nobody knew how to process it. In particular, Jordan's mom withdrew into denial. I later learned that she'd had two early experiences with death that had left her badly scarred and thus doubly resistant to accepting Jordan's condition. Her brother had been killed in a car accident when she was just a teen, and she had been the one who identified his body. The second incident involved her mother, who died from cancer some years later.

Kirsten couldn't join me, since she was just finishing her first year of nursing school and finals were looming. Brittany's mom loved Jordan as much as I did, but she could not arrange to get the time off from work that quickly. As for Brittany, she was in the midst of an emotional crisis of her own. At just shy of seventeen years of age, the terror of Jordan's situation had finally caught up with and overwhelmed her. Watching him nearly suffocate the day before had stunned her, it seemed, and she fell into a state of active panic. Nobody could blame her, but we all realized that, under the circumstances, her presence in Portland would only make things worse.

That left just me.

I started my car and turned onto Oregon State Highway 26, which would lead me across Warm Springs Indian Reservation, then over the hump of the Cascade Mountains and into Portland, Oregon, which bears the nickname the City of Roses, a flower that is perhaps the most classic symbol for love. Physically, I would be making this journey alone. Spiritually, however, I carried with me a wealth of mighty companions the human eye could not detect, though at this particular moment even I did not realize their presence. I have since come to learn that these invisible Teachers are the world's true healers, and while roses may be the symbol of love, these Teachers are Love's essence. In the days to come, they would be making their presence known to me in ways I could never have imagined. They have never left me since.

CHAPTER ELEVEN

A Guide to Meditation

M editation is one of life's rare and purest pleasures, and its beneficial effects on the body are nothing short of astounding. Despite hundreds of studies, researchers still do not understand why meditation has such an enormous positive influence on our health. It is probably the best single activity you can take up for both your physical and emotional well-being. Based on research, regular practitioners can expect around a 50 percent decrease in the chance of developing heart disease — a statistically incredible number considering that heart disease is the number one killer in the United States and many other countries.

The practice has also been shown to reduce the risk of developing cancer by about half, and of suffering from a stroke by approximately 30 percent. It is twice as effective at relieving pain as both acetaminophen and ibuprofen, and it reduces the symptoms of numerous other chronic diseases. If the research is accurate, it may even hold the power to *reverse* heart disease, which is something doctors once thought to be impossible.

It has also been discovered that meditation causes *physical* alterations to the body's structure itself, some at very deep levels. For instance, one study performed by the Benson-Henry Institute for Mind Body Medicine — a top research outfit based out of Massachusetts General Hospital — found that meditative practice alters the way our genes express themselves, affecting more than twenty-two hundred genes at the core of the body's cellular programming. Some of these included genes responsible for overall inflammation in the body, the handling of free radicals, and programmed cell death, all of which play key roles in the development of heart disease, cancer, and aging, among other serious ailments.

Another study conducted by UCLA researchers found that certain parts of the brain responsible for higher human functions, such as positive emotion, decision making, and memory, were enlarged and thickened in individuals who practiced meditation regularly. There is even some emerging data that suggests the practice may increase the number of free stem cells in the blood stream, which are literally the mother of all the body's cells, and as such hold the key to limiting the damage of both stress and aging, processes that are directly linked.

The affect of meditation on the mind is no less astonishing. Practiced perfectly, it has the ability to instantly obliterate the symptoms of depression and anxiety, which are the two most common and profound psychological maladies of our time. According to the Anxiety and Depression Association of America, anxiety is the most common mental disease in the United States, affecting more than forty million people, and the Centers for Disease Control and Prevention's website notes that more than 9 percent of the adult American population suffers from depression (though the real number may be far higher due to the fact that many people who suffer from depression are not even aware of their condition, while others never report it).

Even when practiced imperfectly, meditation can have a profound influence on a person's emotional state and ability to cope with anxiety, depression, and stress. There are numerous reasons for this effect, but one of the most obvious involves the release of a fixation on the past and future. Anxiety almost always involves some projection into the future. The mind either becomes preoccupied with all the possible things that could go wrong in the future or merely overwhelmed with the many tasks and responsibilities that need attending. Depression, on the other hand, is most common in individuals who are apt to live in the past, a tendency that removes us from the joy of the present and often involves a focus on grievances, which is an inherently depressing condition.

The other quality that makes meditation such an attractive alternative to other, less-effective physical and emotional treatments, such as medications, is that the practice has no negative side effects and no cost. You don't have to get a doctor's prescription or drive to the pharmacy to pick up, and pay for, a month's worth of mantras. It's also easy to learn and requires very little time to achieve powerful results.

For all these reasons, and many others, I unreservedly say that meditation is the very best of natural medicine. I highly recommend it to everyone, sick or well, happy or sad. The only catch is that you have to practice regularly. Reading about meditation, discussing it, and thinking about trying it are important steps, but they are not enough. Just as only thinking about exercise won't get you into better physical shape, so too with meditative practice. The key word here is "practice."

Curiously, in the case of meditation, what you are "practicing" involves an intentional attempt at *nondoing*. This is what makes meditation so easy, though many students may at first regard it as difficult. Actually, it requires no effort at all. What makes it seem hard are a student's preconceived notions about it. I used to re-inforce some of these myself, even after I had been teaching the practice for years. Not anymore. Experience has shown me that, given the chance and appropriate instruction, most students natu-rally take to meditation, even those who believe their minds are too busy to meditate. In reality, the mind's natural condition is one of peace and quietness. Thinking requires energy, while meditation is a state of rest. Once you are able to simply relax and let go, your mind will automatically shift into the meditative space. Therefore you don't actually have to do anything at all to meditate.

Imagine taking a raft out into a gently flowing river. Every-day life for most of us is akin to trying to paddle a raft upstream against the current. Meditation, on the other hand, is like allowing the raft and the river to carry you along with no effort required on your part, thus leaving you free to enjoy the wonder of the jour-ney, the beauty of the land and water that surrounds you.

This is not to say that you won't experience resistance to med-itation. Everyone does to some degree. If you ever feel frustrated with your practice, just remember that Buddha had trouble with meditation! But also keep in mind that this resistance is not spe-cifically due to meditative practice itself. Resistance, in any form, actually represents a struggle against the state of *being*, which is merely a state of mind in which you allow the current of life to carry your raft. You are already on a raft. Of that, you have no choice. That is life — a raft on a river. The only true choice that is ours to make involves whether to struggle against the current, a process that is exhausting and at times terrifying, or to relax and flow with it, an act requiring no effort whatsoever.

Paddling upstream, or trying to guide your raft in one direc-tion or another, merely represents the need to cling to the ego state through mental projections into the past and future. As such it implies a lack of trust in the universe. It is a way of asserting that

you must be in control of your life and direct your own destiny —
as if you know better than Life what you need and which direction
you should go. Of course, we are bound to do this to some degree.
Indeed, we are all asked to make occasional, minor adjustments as
we proceed down the river of life. Meditation does not ask you to
have perfect, unfailing faith in the River. It merely asks that you
set aside brief periods of time in which you cease your efforts and
your struggle and surrender entirely to the will of the current.

Most people find developing a meditative practice enjoyable.
The trick is not to try too hard or go into the practice with unreal-
istic expectations, which are bound to lead to disappointment. At
first you will probably feel a simple sense of peace, inner quietness,
and perhaps a feeling of safety, as if you have been wrapped in a
warm cocoon, or perhaps like you are floating. You have probably had occasions when you have touched this space already:
times when you were just relaxing and enjoying the moment,
brief periods when you slipped beyond your sense of limited self-
perception. Just about everyone has felt this, though they may not
have realized what was occurring. Some people experience this
transcendent state while participating in sports, hiking, reading
a book, practicing yoga, exercising, or just sitting by a river or
the sea, listening to the sound of the water. Anything that draws
your attention to the here and now or that lends itself to quietness
can be a trigger. These moments happen spontaneously when we
release our defenses and stop struggling against the direction life
is carrying us. The only difference between such spontaneous
glimpses and organized practice is that during meditation you *intentionally* attempt to access this awareness.

What Is Meditation?

This may seem like a simple question, and it is. Most students new
to meditation ask it, and yet the answers they receive, even from

well-meaning instructors, are not always particularly helpful. For some reason this question provokes a great variety of complex or vague responses, rather than clarity and simplicity, which, to me, is the heart of meditation. Ask a dozen meditation teachers this simple-seeming question and you may receive a dozen different responses. Some teachers may reply with silence or simply shrug their shoulders, implying that meditation is a mystery that words cannot answer; another teacher might reply mysteriously, "How can one define in words a practice that is designed to lead the student beyond words?"

In a sense these answers are valid. In another sense, at least for the new meditation student, they aren't particularly helpful.

To understand meditation, the first thing to realize is that there is a difference between the *techniques* of meditation and the *experience* of meditation. Most techniques are easily explained. For instance, the practice of zazen simply involves counting your breaths while trying to relax. On the other hand, the experience of meditation is not so easily explained and is usually the source of any confusion. Experiences are often hard to describe to those who have never had them. For example, how would you describe a sunset blazing on the horizon over the Pacific Ocean to someone who had been born blind and had never seen the sun, the horizon, or the ocean? How would you relate to a deaf person the emotions sparked by the rising and falling of notes and the blending of melodies that make up a beautiful song? These would be exceedingly challenging tasks no matter how great a sculptor of words one happened to be. Further, lacking the sense in question, how accurate would the blind or deaf person's mental picture be, especially held up next to the reality of the experience?

So it is with meditation. Teachers who point out that meditation cannot be adequately described are correct. If you have never meditated before, you will have to practice it for yourself in order to form your own direct understanding of what it is and how it feels. But what *can* be explained is the *direction* you need to proceed, along with the conditions you need to meet, in order to discover that experience.

The Island of Meditation

Picture yourself standing at the edge of a lake. In the middle of the lake is an island. Along the shoreline are a number of boats. The island in the middle represents the experience of meditation. I cannot tell you, in words, much about this island, other than that you are really going to enjoy it. It is truly lovely. You want to get there.

The boats on the shore represent the various techniques of meditative practice, such as zazen, mantras, mindfulness, and so on. Each boat is a little different. Some may be faster but more difficult to handle, less stable, or harder to steer. Some move across the lake more slowly, but perhaps are more comfortable. Also, each student is a little different, with differing personalities, backgrounds, and obstacles to reaching the island of meditation. Therefore, the boat that best suits one person may not work so well for another. This is why I suggest new students try out several techniques to gauge which feels most natural.

While I may not be able to adequately describe what the island itself is like, I can help you learn how best to manage the various boats. The other thing I can do is suggest which direction you should aim your boat, just as sailors use compasses and GPS systems to guide them across the world's oceans. Here, then, are the coordinates of the island of meditation.

Coordinate 1: The Island of Meditation Exists in the Now

The present moment is the center of meditative awareness. Think of it this way: The past is like the wake a boat leaves behind as it crosses the water; the wake is not the boat itself and it has nothing to do with you. It is the result of your passage, but it has no effects and it dissipates rapidly. Similarly, the future looks forward into the unseen distance over the horizon. Doing so deadens your awareness of the immediate present, mentally removing you from what *is*. In a sense, when you think about either the past or future, neither of which actually exist, you are seeing what is not there and are therefore hallucinating.

I grew up in Southern California, and as a kid I spent many weekends combing the California coastline in search of waves to surf. I didn't realize it back then, but surfing was probably my first major exposure to meditation. The act lends itself to present-moment awareness. It naturally quiets the mind, even when you are just sitting around, bobbing along the surface of the sea, waiting for the next set of waves to arrive. Somehow the motion of the water, the energy of the sea, and the mighty expanse of the horizon all work together to draw the mind into the present. And when you do take off on a wave and sync with the phenomenal energy it contains, the whole world seems to vanish as you enter what feels like a parallel universe that only surfers know exists. In it the entire universe suddenly consists of only you, your board, and the swell unfurling around you.

When I started teaching meditation, I often used the expression *surfing the now* to help students understand the practice. If you paddle out into the ocean on a surfboard, you need to be in just the right spot to catch a wave. If you paddle too far out to sea, the waves are only unformed swells, impossible to catch. If you are too close to shore, the waves become too steep to ride, and they may break immediately in front of you or right on top of you, which can be dangerous.

In order to catch a wave, you have to find the sweet spot where the swells are just beginning to steepen and become breaking waves. The same is true of surfing the now. When you meditate, try to put all thoughts of the past out of your mind. Don't think about anything that has occurred in the past, whether it happened a year ago, a month ago, or even just an instant before. Try to let every moment be fresh and new, and keep your mind as clean of old thoughts as possible. To dwell on the past during meditation is like positioning yourself too close to shore while surfing; you will be stuck in the turbulence of the breaking surf.

Likewise, do not allow your thoughts to drift into the future, whether these thoughts are pleasant or negative. When you mentally wander into future concerns during meditation, you drift too far out to sea. You become hypnotized by the distant horizon, dreaming of what's to be or not to be. Then all the best waves will pass beneath you and you won't even notice. Even minuscule shifts into the past or future will reduce the depth of your meditation.

The now is always with you, arising with every new instant of your life, just as the waves of the ocean do. It is unfolding this very instant, even as you read this. The question always is, *where are you?* As you release your focus on the past and future, you will sense the swell of pure being awakening and steepening within you, and you will begin to understand the spacious joy that comes from connecting with its energy and balancing on its crest as you race across the unfolding and unfathomable majesty of the now.

Coordinate 2: The Island of Meditation Exists Within You

The island of meditation is not something that your physical eye can see or that your hands can touch. It is invisible, and it exists within you, although its peace and light can certainly be reflected in the outside world. This is exactly what Jesus meant when he told his followers (in Luke 17:21), "The Kingdom of God is within you." The island of meditation *is* the Kingdom of God, and because it is within us, it is very close to each of us indeed.

The only reason most people are unaware of the island's presence is because we are all too busy focusing on the outside world, which lies in the exact opposite direction. We are looking in the wrong place.

During meditation, then, part of the objective is to switch the direction of your attention from the world outside to the world within. This is why I usually recommend finding a quiet place to meditate where you can close your eyes and focus on the journey into inner space as deeply as possible. To the best of your ability, loosen your grip on all thoughts relating to everything connected to the outside world, once again whether those thoughts are positive or negative. Forget about the world and everything in it while you meditate, no matter how important your thoughts seem to be. Don't worry, the world is not going anywhere. It will still be around when you are done meditating, along with all the things you think are important.

As simple as the practice of releasing your thoughts about the world may seem, you are bound to find yourself deeply rewarded by the practice, for while the circumstances of your life may not change during meditation, your view of your circumstances *will*. Through meditation you will eventually come to understand the greatness of the world that lies within you and, by contrast, the littleness of the physical world, which most of us take far too seriously. You may also realize how insignificant our worldly troubles really are, and how petty are our judgments, though they do lead to the violence and savagery that marks the human race as the world's most destructive species.

Meditation is like a tiny star, a pinprick of light, that appears like a light of hope in the darkness of this violent and sad world. It may, perhaps, seem to be only a faint star at first, but it contains a power far greater than the world's darkness because it comes from our Native Home, and with its coming it reminds us that we are not creatures of time and space, and violence and hatred, but limitless, omniscient beings of strength and innocence. Every time you sit down to meditate another star will light your mind, until eventually the darkness will give way to dusk, and you will one day open your inner eye in astonishment as you discover that a universe of light exists inside you. And then, at last, you will understand why this process is called enlightenment.

Coordinate 3: The Island of Meditation Exists in Stillness and Quietness

Finally, when you meditate, do your best to remain as still as possible and let your thoughts grow quiet and peaceful. This doesn't mean that you can't occasionally readjust your sitting position if you feel the need. Fighting against this urge, and struggle in general, is antithetical to the practice, and so it is best avoided. When necessary, simply shift your sitting posture without making a big deal out of it.

In general, when it comes to handling your thoughts during meditation, try to keep your mind focused on thoughts that generate a sense of safety, peace, and quietness because the island of mediation is a place of tranquility. Turbulent thoughts will interfere with your experience and reduce your awareness of the island. However, as with attempting to remain still, it is best not to fight against the thoughts that come into your mind even if they seem unpleasant. Whatever their form, let them arise as they will, but don't cling to any of them. If it helps, imagine them as clouds in the sky that are just passing through your consciousness. You will see clouds of many shapes, colors, and sizes, but whatever their appearance try not to allow them to trap your attention. They are just clouds; nothing important. When you sit down to meditate, resign yourself to simply watching your thoughts come and go while remaining unattached to any pattern in particular. You are not the clouds; you are the *presence* observing the clouds.

How to Sit

Some meditation teachers suggest a strict sitting posture for practicing, but I've never found that perfect posture makes much of a difference. Ram Dass, the great spiritual teacher and author, once told a story about attending a Buddhist retreat during which the teacher walked around whacking students with a stick if their backs were not perfectly straight, shoulders pulled back, and chins tucked in so as to elongate the rear of the neck, which is a classic meditation posture. In my view, there are far more important matters when it comes to your practice than how you choose to sit. With this in mind, there are a few key points to consider.

1. Sit up when you meditate. Lying down may increase drowsiness and withdrawal, a common problem during meditation, especially in beginners. Despite appearances, meditation is not a state of passive withdrawal toward sleep, but a progressive *increase* in awareness.

2. You may sit on a chair or sofa with your feet flat on the floor, or sit on a cushion on the ground or on your bed with your legs crossed in front of you. Alternatively, flexible students may prefer to cross one or both ankles over the opposing thighs, adopting what are commonly referred to as the half-lotus and lotus positions, respectively. There are also specialty meditation pillows and benches, which are available online and through spiritual supply stores.

3. However you choose to sit, keep your back comfortably straight. Avoid slouching, which increases muscle strain and may interfere with deep meditation.

4. Rest your hands wherever they fall naturally, whether in your

lap, along your legs, or on the ground or seat beside you. You may cup them atop one another or not, lace your fingers together or not, and the palms may be positioned either up or down as you prefer.

5. Use pillows or cushions as needed, placed either below or behind you (or both) to improve comfort.

6. You can meditate with some form of support behind your back (such as a wall or chair back), or with no support, whichever is most comfortable. Many students begin by using some form of back support but eventually, as the muscles of the back adapt and strengthen, find it best to sit freely with nothing pressed against the back.

It may take you some experimentation and practice to figure out which sitting position is most comfortable for you, as well as to get used to remaining still. This is normal, but don't get frustrated. Over time your body will adapt and soon enough you will hardly even notice your body while you are meditating.

How Long, Where, and When Should You Meditate?

Strictly speaking, there is no bad place or time to meditate. I have practiced on the bus, as a passenger in cars, while waiting for appointments, and during breaks at my desk. For especially busy people, any spare moment can make a great time to squeeze in a brief meditation. You don't even necessarily need to close your eyes. Simply relaxing, turning within, and tuning in to your breath, or focusing on a silent mantra, can certainly be done with the eyes open in any environment.

With that said, it is still helpful to establish a regular time for practicing during which you can withdraw from the world in a significant way and devote your full attention to your meditation without distractions. I suggest you choose a regular space and time that are convenient and relatively quiet.

Some people choose to meditate in their bedroom, since this is often the only personal space available. This is a fine choice. However, if you do have an extra room, or even a corner of a room, it is helpful to set up a space specifically devoted to your practice. The theory is that over time the environment becomes infused with quiet energy, which helps you to go deeper into meditation more rapidly. You can design this space however suits your taste and beliefs. If it inspires you, you might, for example, set up some sort of an altar, with candles, incense, pictures or drawings of spiritual teachers, sacred books, and any other items that elicit a sense of peace and holiness.

Some people enjoy the sound of bells, chimes, or background music while they meditate; if you wish, place a stereo or speakers in the space as well. There are hundreds of meditation albums available through specialty spiritual stores and the Internet. Many mainstream stores carry a selection of nature sounds and meditation CDs, which also work great for meditation, and of course, most music and dozens of apps can be downloaded onto electronic devices.

As for when you should meditate, I suggest you practice as soon as possible after waking up, and then once more before going to bed. It is helpful to meditate in the morning before you begin your day. This grounds you in a state of general peace and sets the tone for a tranquil day ahead. Remember when you were in grade school and your teacher took the role? When your name was called, you were expected to raise your hand to indicate that you were present in class. Morning meditations serve a similar purpose. They are a way of reminding yourself that you are present, accounted for, and aware that you are in the classroom called Earth School and are ready to begin the day's lessons consciously.

Likewise, it is important to check back in with your Teacher in the evening and make an effort to expel whatever stress and negative emotions you may have accumulated during the day. I call this process *putting out the garbage before bed*. Expunging the day's stressors at night will help you sleep more deeply and get the most out of your rest. It is also an excellent way to ensure that you are not accumulating toxic emotional baggage over time.

Regarding the length of your meditations, this depends on you, how busy your life is, and how comfortable you are with the practice. Traditionally, teachers once suggested very long meditations, but that thinking has started to shift. When students attempt to meditate for long periods of time, they often find themselves wildly restless to such a degree that they are not really meditating at all; they are merely sitting with their eyes closed while actively thinking. For this reason, most beginners should meditate for short periods while concentrating as deeply as possible. A focused, twenty-minute session is more helpful than an hour of restless thinking. In general, to begin, aim for about fifteen or twenty minutes. If you find this time to be too long, reduce the amount to as little as five or ten minutes, or even less if necessary. Deepak Chopra once suggested that if you have time to brush your teeth in the morning, you have time to meditate. On the other hand, if you discover that twenty minutes pass with little sense of strain and you are still enjoying your experience, by all means increase the amount of time.

One interesting fact in this regard is that much of the research on meditation's benefits has studied relatively short meditation periods, often in the twenty-minute range twice daily. Meditation appears to produce benefits with very little effort and time invested. Also, many of these studies used participants who were new to the practice. Apparently, it does not take long for meditation to begin affecting you. For instance, in the Benson-Henry

Institute study cited above that found that meditation alters our genes, three groups were studied. One group consisted of experienced meditators, the second group was made up of new practitioners, and the third group was people who did not meditate at all, either before or during the study. Compared to nonmeditators, experienced practitioners showed differences in more than twenty-two hundred genes, and new practitioners displayed differences in about sixteen hundred genes.

Once again, the most important thing is to practice regularly. Even if you feel you aren't getting much from the experience of meditation, your body knows otherwise.

Before You Begin: Get Settled and Relaxed

There are many forms of meditation. In this book I introduce just a few. However, all begin in the same way. In each meditation style that follows, the first step is to "get settled and relaxed." Here is a simple, foolproof way of preparing yourself for meditation:

1. Choose a relatively quiet place and time where you can be alone. Turn off your phone, close the door, and dim the lights if you like.
2. Set a timer or a gentle alarm to keep track of time, or just briefly open your eyes and check the clock as needed.
3. Sit comfortably and close your eyes.
4. Take a few deep, slow breaths, breathing in through your nose and out through your mouth. Be sure to allow air to fill the lower lobes of your lungs so that your belly pops out just a little, like a pregnant woman. Also, exhale fully so that all the air, and waste, is completely expelled from your body. Deep breathing triggers a natural relaxation response. It is a great way to start your meditation. After taking three or four breaths in this manner, let your breathing return to normal.

5. Now intentionally focus on relaxing your body. Begin with your toes and feet; next relax your calf muscles and thighs; then move onto your hips and lower back. Try to feel as if the tension and stress stored in your muscles is dissipating into the air. When the lower half of your body is sufficiently relaxed, let this sense of restfulness move upward through your torso and into your chest and upper back, like a warm current expanding upward through your body. As you release the tension stored in your shoulders you may feel them sag just a little, and your arms may in turn dip. This is fine. Just let all sense of tension go and concentrate on relaxing completely. Next, let this feeling spread down your arms and through your hands, and even into your fingers. Finally, sense it moving up and over your head and through your face, including your scalp, brow, cheeks, and jaw line.

When you are done, there should be no sense of tension remaining in your body. The whole sequence need only take two or three minutes, and it should leave you feeling as if you have been wrapped in a warm cocoon of light, in which you feel safe, quiet, and perfectly at peace.

Mantra

Mantra is one of the most common styles of the practice, as well as one of the most effective and easiest to learn, and there are numerous mantras to choose from. A mantra is simply a word, sound, sentence, or series of sentences that is repeatedly spoken aloud or thought silently during meditation. Mantras serve a couple of purposes. For one, they occupy the ego mind while you are attempting to relax and allow the state of being to surface into awareness. The mantra gives you a repetitive thought to focus on, which helps you avoid straying into random thought patterns (or *thought webs,* as I call them, due to their tendency to entrap the student's attention). Mantras can also instill a sense of quietness, safety, and peace.

First, select a mantra to use. For this exercise we will use the mantra "Peace, calm, still." You can find many more mantras in meditation books (such as my book *The Power of Stillness*) and online.

1. Get settled and relaxed.

2. Spend a few minutes enjoying this sense of restfulness, then, when you are ready, begin repeating your mantra. For this particular form of mantra, repeat one word during every exhalation. So, as you breathe out, think, silently to yourself, the word "peace." Then, during your next out-breath, think, "calm." Finally, with your third exhalation, silently focus on the word "still." Continue to repeat the mantra every time you breathe out for the duration of the meditation, starting over again from "peace."

3. Many thoughts will occur to you as you practice in this way. At times you will forget to repeat the mantra all together. Minutes may pass as you become lost in some pattern of random thoughts. Don't struggle or allow yourself to become frustrated when this happens. It's a normal part of the process. Do try, however, to view your thoughts impartially, as if they were nothing more than clouds passing overhead. Let them come and let them go, and whenever you remember, recall your attention to the practice of repeating the mantra.

4. In addition to the repetitions of the mantra, every time you exhale you may also find it helpful to focus on the sensation of relaxing your body. Imagine that no matter how relaxed you become, your body is always capable of relaxing just a little deeper. Let go and surrender fully to this sense of tranquility. If it helps, remind yourself that you are perfectly safe during

this practice. Even if you already feel safe, you may benefit from reminding yourself anyway. You can go as deeply into meditation as you like and you will only experience peace and a growing sense of joy and release.

5. After you are done, open your eyes and sit quietly for a few minutes, allowing the sense of restfulness and calm to remain with you. This final step is something I suggest you do after every meditation, regardless of the form being used.

Zazen

Zazen is a Zen practice that is similar to mantra meditation, except instead of repeating words or sentences, you count your breaths.

1. Get settled and relaxed.
2. Once you are ready to begin, start counting your out-breaths. So, as you breathe out, think to yourself, silently, "one," and focus on relaxing your body as instructed above. During your next out-breath think, "two," then "three," and so on, until you reach "ten," at which point begin counting again from "one."
3. Repeat this cycle for the duration of the meditation. As thoughts occur to you and you find yourself forgetting to count your breaths, try to let thoughts pass unobstructed, and return your attention to counting, starting again from "one." Anytime you become lost in thought, or confused as to what number you were on, begin again from "one."
4. Afterward, sit quietly for a few minutes.

Mindfulness

To be mindful merely means to "pay attention to." Mindfulness is a simple meditative practice that can be performed anywhere, at any time. There is virtually no circumstance that is not suitable. You can even practice mindfulness with your eyes open and while engaged in conversations and physical activities. The most common form is mindfulness of the breath. The process of becoming aware of the immediate sense of your breath draws the mind away from thoughts about past and future and centers it on the present. In fact, a part of the power of both mantra and zazen lie in their ability to sync your attention with the respiratory cycle.

1. Get settled and relaxed.
2. When you are ready, place your attention on your breath by becoming subtly aware of the passage of air into and out of your lungs. You might focus on the sensation of your chest rising and falling, or on the feeling of air where you feel it entering your body, such as across the upper lip or at the threshold of the nostrils. Notice how the air is cooler as it enters the body and subtly warmer as it exits.
3. Keep your awareness concentrated on the respiratory cycle. When your mind wanders, remember to let your distracting thoughts pass by without engaging you, and pull your attention gently, but firmly, back to the breath.
4. During this practice, also attempt to be aware of the state of pure *being* that underlies the exercise. Try to experience yourself as the presence that exists independent of your thoughts, body, and actions. You are not them, and they are not you; you are the observer behind them, and your life is not dependent on the body or its actions and thoughts.
5. Afterward, sit quietly for a few minutes.

Third-Eye Meditation

The so-called third eye is a part of the chakra system, which traditionally includes seven sacred points that run through the body from the crown of the head to the base of the spine. The third eye is located approximately between the eyebrows. Focusing on this point during meditation is thought to deepen the meditative experience. To practice third-eye meditation, train your attention at the point between your eyebrows while you practice any of the above meditations, such as a mantra, or simply keep your awareness centered there and sit silently, letting your thoughts come and go without engaging you. As usual, when your mind wanders, return your focus to the practice. If it helps, you might imagine mentally "pressing" your attention against your forehead rather than trying to specifically target the third eye itself.

Meditation may seem challenging at first, but with practice and dedication, it gets easier until one day you will no longer understand why you ever found it hard. Whichever form you choose, remain focused on relaxing and letting go. Noneffort is the key that makes meditation so easy. Remember, whether meditation feels like a joy or a chore to you at any given time, even when you feel you are not getting anything from the practice, you are still benefiting whether you realize it or not. Difficulty in concentrating won't diminish meditation's many gifts to you. Only failing to practice will.

CHAPTER TWELVE

The Art of Visualization

Visualization is really a form of meditation. It has special applications as a healing method, however, and using it for this purpose differs slightly from the more traditional meditative practices. For this reason, we will consider it separately.

It has been estimated that the average person uses only 10 percent or less of the capabilities inherent in the human mind. My guess is that this number is considerably lower. Our thoughts are so scattered and unfocused that most of us scarcely harness anywhere close to 10 percent of our mind's full capacity. This is unfortunate, for focus, desire, and belief are the holy trinity of forces that shape our destiny. When you concentrate with genuine desire on the things you believe you are fully capable of manifesting into your life, you become an active, conscious participant in the creation of your experience. For those readers who have studied this teaching in books like *Law of Attraction* and *The Secret*, you probably already understand this concept. If not, it is something every human being who wishes to live a life of empowerment must master. When concentration, desire, and belief align, miracles become possible.

Focus

In my late teens and early twenties before I had kids, I used to ride a motorcycle. I knew it could be dangerous, but I didn't care. It was fun, cheap transportation, and I was young. Back then I didn't even bother to wear a helmet, I never received any formal rider's training, and I didn't even have a motorcycle license. In reality, I didn't know the first thing about riding, though of course I thought I did.

Fortunately, I never had an accident, but I did have a few close calls. After my first daughter was born, I joined the real world and figured I'd better make an effort to stick around the planet a while. I sold my bike and bought a four-door compact car, and I always wore my seatbelt. Many years later, well after my girls were fully grown, I decided to take up riding again when gas prices skyrocketed to four bucks a gallon. This time, however, the first thing I did was go take a rider's safety course. The class was a fantastic experience. I never thought I could learn so much about riding a motorcycle, and riding life, all at once. In fact, the class's very first lesson turned out to be one that could be applied to life in many arenas, and which I will remember forever:

Always look in the direction you want to go!

As it turns out, a motorcycle is not steered by your arms and your body weight so much as with your eyes and your focus. Where you look is where you will go. Focus on the potholes in the road, the cars that suddenly veer in front of you, or the trees along the side of the street, and you become an accident waiting to happen. Suddenly, those close shaves I'd had as a kid while riding my little red 305 cc Kawasaki made sense.

Also as it turns out, this principle applies to the general hazards of life, no matter what topic we are considering: focus on your troubles, and you will likely find those troubles multiplying and expanding; concentrate on lack, and you will probably create more deprivation in your life; obsess about disease, and illness may gradually become a way of life for you.

Have you ever seen one of those funny videos of a new snow skier heading down a bunny slope for the first time? He starts out at the top of a gentle hill that has been completely cleared of obstacles...except, perhaps, for one skinny little tree at the bottom of the slope, way off to the side. As he sets off, you know there's no way he's going to hit the tree because he has the entire empty, treeless space in front of him. Yet, because he's looking right at the one obstacle in his path in the hopes of avoiding it, he somehow manages, incredibly, to angle right for it, all the way down the hill, until he crashes straight into it.

Why does this happen? In one word — *focus.* Just as you can't steer a motorcycle with your body, neither can you steer skis, or a bicycle, or life with your body.

The moral of this story is that if you want to attract success, happiness, and health into your life while avoiding the trees, you must train your mind to focus on what you wish to have, not on the things you want to avoid. Do not fixate on the obstacles in your path unless you want to be drawn into them. Instead, when trees and potholes pop up — and they will! — you must train yourself to concentrate on the path *around* them. In the context of healing, this means you should avoid filling your mind with images and thoughts about everything that is wrong with you, or that could go wrong in the future. Why not obsess over all that is *right* with your mind and body? Cultivate a sense of anticipation that steers you toward good health and increasing strength, vitality, and happiness. In other words, focus on the positive, not on the negative. Make it a habit, and remember that doing so is nothing more complicated than a choice. Do not delude yourself into believing otherwise.

Desire

Now that you understand the importance of focus, the next thing to clarify is the role desire plays in shaping your life. A general guideline about desire states:

> That which you truly want, in the depths of your heart, is that which will manifest in the circumstances of your life.

Now, this rule doesn't necessarily apply to specifics, and it is heavily influenced by what you believe you *deserve*. For instance, you may tell yourself that you want a million dollars, but that is just the *form* of your desire. What you are really asking for is financial security and freedom. Also, the words you use don't necessarily matter. Perhaps you tell yourself you want to be rich, but if you don't believe you deserve financial stability, it's never going to happen. Essentially you are lying to yourself. Your mouth is saying one thing, but your heart is singing an entirely different tune. Yet it is only the heart that the universe listens to because it is only the heart that is incapable of lying. Words, on the other hand, are easily manipulated.

Because of the profound affect your desires have on your life, if you want to be in control of your destiny, you need to get ultra clear on what it is you truly want, as well as ultra clear on what it is you believe you deserve. In order to do this, you have to get real with yourself, which means you need to become supremely open and honest, even if the truth turns out to be less than appealing. Open your awareness to what you authentically believe you want out of life, whatever it happens to be. This is the only way to clear room for change. Make an honest and detailed appraisal of the things you truly long for, and then ask yourself if you also believe you deserve those things. If it turns out you don't like the things and circumstances your heart longs for, change your goals; and if you find you do like them but you don't believe you deserve them, it's time to upgrade your sense of self-worth.

Honesty requires courage, and what you find may surprise you as you dig through the various motivations and hopes that populate your consciousness. Most people suffer from lowly self-images, and very few of us aspire to the heights of which we are capable. If you discover this is true for you, I urge you to challenge any and all false, self-defeating opinions of who you are and what you are capable of achieving. There is no question about it — you have talents that you are not even aware exist, and those talents are lying dormant, unappreciated and unused while you fail to seize your potential.

So focus is like the steering wheel of life, and desire is the engine that fuels our journey. Ultimately you need to be in control of both these forces, or your life will essentially be stuck on autopilot mode, and you may perceive your life to be chaotic and out of control.

Belief

Belief is the king of all the forces that shape our lives. It can be a limiter or a liberator, depending on the particular belief. Our capabilities are limited by nothing more than what we personally believe we can accomplish. It is not enough to want the best out of life; you must also believe that your goals are really possible to achieve. This is why a patient must believe he or she is capable of healing in order to do so. The need to believe in your ability to meet your goals goes beyond healing, however. It is applicable to all areas of your life, from professional goals to relationships to physical capabilities, and beyond. Students must believe they are capable of passing a test if they wish to succeed; doctors must trust that their patients can be successfully treated; business executives must have faith in themselves to close the deals that build their companies. If you don't think you can do it, neither will the universe — because you *are* the universe. The life Force that makes up your own life is the same Force that shaped the cosmos. This Force can neither be limited nor prevented from extending; it can only be directed.

The message here is simply that you must sculpt and direct your beliefs carefully and consciously. If you believe life is bleak and bad and filled with darkness, pain, and disaster, so will it seem to be. If you think life is a place of hope and happiness, and you believe you were born into the world to add to the abundance of joy where there is joy, and to bring light and healing where there is a need for it, this happy state will become your reality.

Whether or not you are aware of the formula of creation, it is true, it is always in force, and it adds up to your destiny. One: Focus on what you want, and not what you do not want. Two: Make sure your efforts are in line with your *authentic* desires. Three: Believe in your ability to achieve your goals and shape your life, and trust in the universe to help you along the way. Write this formula down, cut it out, and tape it to your bathroom mirror or on your fridge so you see it every morning before you walk out the door:

Focus + Desire + Belief = Destiny

The Art of Visualization

Visualization is a tool that can help you consciously direct these three forces. It is a way of clarifying what it is you want to manifest in your life, bringing it into clear, mental focus, and holding it there. It is based on the notion that *what becomes real in the mind becomes real in the flesh*.

This means that if you are able to see something in your mind first, clearly, and hold your intention to bring that something into your life without allowing negative beliefs and contradictory desires to interfere, you will vastly increase the odds of attracting it into your physical circumstances.

In this book we focus on visualizations specifically designed for healing, but these same basic techniques can be applied to any aspect of your life. Successful business executives have been known to close their eyes and visualize themselves sealing that perfect, once-in-a-lifetime deal. Many athletes also practice visualization in order to increase their performance. For instance, a runner might close his or her eyes and sit for a few minutes before a race and imagine running in fluid strides ahead of everyone else and crossing the finish line in first place.

Of course, our health is far more important than money or a trophy, which, in the grand scheme of life, are meaningless. The following exercises stimulate the healing process by activating and focusing the power of the mind. Whenever possible, patients may wish to apply these visual exercises while actively receiving any medical treatments or immediately after taking medication. Applied with deep concentration, these exercises can provide a powerful boost to physical treatments.

Healing Light Visualization

I led Jordan through the following visualization exercise while he was actively receiving his targeted chemo treatments. It makes a particularly potent supplement to medical treatment, helping the patient to amplify the effects of medications and other forms of therapy. Ideally, apply it while receiving treatment or immediately afterward.

1. Get settled and relaxed.
2. Imagine a sphere of golden light resting near your core, like a miniature sun, in the area of your heart chakra. Now imagine

that this ball of light represents pure, healing Source energy. It brings balance and healing to every cell it touches.

3. Picture the light growing a little brighter each time you breathe in, increasing in intensity. Then, as you exhale, see it flowing from your chest through the rest of your body, moving from your heart down to the tips of your fingers; through your torso, and into your legs, feet, and toes; and upward into your head. Repeat this visualization with every respiratory cycle: breathing in, the light grows brighter, breathing out, it flows through your body.

4. As the light passes through you, imagine that it is healing every function, organ, and cell in your body. Try not to think of it as *destroying* the disease so much as healing it. It is better to focus on positive visuals rather than destructive imagery.

5. Practice this visualization for fifteen minutes no more than once a day for a maximum of one week at a stretch. It should not be overused, but you are encouraged to supplement it with other meditations. If there is a particular area in your body in need of healing, you may focus primarily on it for the last five minutes of the exercise, visualizing *all* of the Source energy flowing from your heart directly to the area in question, infusing it with vitality, energy, and healing.

Healing with the Masters Visualization

It has been said that a truly enlightened being never dies. When the moment comes to leave the earth, they do so consciously and with intention. Instead of dying, they enter a state known in the Hindu tradition as *mahasamadhi*, which is a master's final, conscious exit from the body. Afterward, the master becomes a fully liberated Teacher — free from all limitations. Of course, you do not need to convert to Hinduism to make this transition. It is equally possible for anyone, whether you follow a religious tradition or not.

It has also been said that such Beings are always available to help those of us who are still learning in the classrooms of Earth School. All we have to do is call upon Them for help when we are in need, and then become quiet enough to hear Their answer. The second portion of this procedure is the tricky part. The problem is the voice of the ego is so dominant in most of our minds that it drowns out the voice of the Masters, who are very gentle and quiet in Their ways, despite Their limitless power. Learning to become quiet and at peace even in the midst of crisis, then, is essential.

The following visual exercise is designed to assist you in opening up to the healing energy of these Great Teachers. I first began to sense Their presence in me while Jordan was in the ICU in Portland. It is quite a startling experience to realize that you are not alone in the universe, and that you are connected to an entire constellation of life, which includes healers such as Christ, Buddha, and others. These Beings are not distant from us. Indeed, they are one with us.

These Healers live within you, too, and there is nothing They cannot accomplish. In my opinion, it was They, not I — nor anyone else — who were ultimately responsible for Jordan's recovery.

Perform the following exercise as you would any meditation:

1. Get settled and relaxed.
2. Begin by imagining yourself sitting with a Master Healer. This may be a well-known spiritual teacher, such as Jesus, Buddha, Krishna, or Muhammad, or some other great teacher of peace and healing. Or you can simply imagine a field of glowing, golden Light.
3. Picture yourself seated facing this Being. Take a minute to regard Them. Notice how still They are. How quiet Their eyes are. How peaceful and filled with light and holiness.... This Being's presence is a thing of immense power and entrancing beauty.

4. Then, silently in your thoughts, with as much conviction as possible, speak the following words:

Give me your blessing, Great Teacher.
Let me realize that You and I are one.
Your holiness is my holiness.
Your peace is my peace.
Your strength is my strength.
Your body is my body.
Your mind is my mind.
I have no life apart from You.
We are one.
Therefore, I must be healed.

If you have trouble remembering this prayer, open your eyes in order to read it. Then, repeat it slowly, several times, letting the words sink deeply into your thoughts.

5. Next, with your eyes closed, imagine your Teacher placing Their hand atop the crown of your head. Sense Their energy moving into your body, visualizing it as a golden, healing Light. Your thoughts are quiet and you feel intensely tranquil. Let this sense of quietude enwrap you fully, and allow yourself to totally surrender. Release your ego, let go of fear, and free yourself from any awareness of your body. Imagine that in place of your body is now the self-same Light that was a gift from your Teacher — as if your entire being is composed only of Light. How can Light be sick?

6. Remain focused on this state of direct communion for several minutes or longer.

7. After you are done, open your eyes and sit quietly for a few minutes.

CHAPTER THIRTEEN

The Intensive Care Unit

The drive to Portland took three and a half winding hours, which passed in a fog. Along the way, my panic evolved into a dull sense of numbness, which is a classic emotional defense. Some situations are so overwhelming the mind just shuts down, and you find yourself operating on autopilot. This was one of those instances. The day was clear, and the drive a beautiful one, but I don't recall a single mile of it.

Once I reached Portland, locating the hospital at Oregon Health & Science University (OHSU), and then finding Jordan himself, proved to be difficult. OHSU's hospital commands a stellar view from a broad hillside overlooking Portland's city center and the Willamette River far below. Yet despite the behemoth facility's size, it is a challenging place to find. The only road up to its lofty perch happens to be a tiny street in a complex section of the city. Furthermore, the hospital is just one part of a giant medical complex that includes Doernbecher Children's Hospital, the Portland VA Medical Center, and Shriners Hospital for Children. If you ever visit similar facilities, be sure to allow extra time just to find your way around. Any way you can reduce stress when dealing with a medical crisis, you should, and this is certainly a common, albeit minor, stressor.

When I finally found Jordan in the intensive care unit, he was surrounded by hospital staff. Though he had arrived by plane several hours ahead of me, he was still in the process of being admitted. It was a frantic rush. He had already received a battery of blood work and an MRI, which is a full body scan that utilizes a strong magnetic field, radio signals, and a sophisticated computer system to provide a detailed, interior view of the patient's body. Jordan was still on oxygen, an IV drip fed meds into his arm, and electrodes taped to his chest were continuously monitoring his heart rate, respiration, and blood oxygen level.

Jordan was still waiting on the MRI results. For those dealing with the modern medical system, be prepared to have your patience tested and tested again. Patients and their families do *a lot* of waiting. I suggest you use such moments cultivating mindfulness, which is the only way to reduce anxiety in such critical situations. The act of "waiting" itself is a major contributor to the misery so often reported by patients and their loved ones, but it is really only a mental mode.

The rooms in the intensive care unit at OHSU are different than most hospital rooms I've been in. They are intended to be functional, not comfortable. Beyond a chair and a television, creature comforts are few. The unit is not set up for long-term stays. Most patients either quickly recover enough to be transferred to other wings of the hospital or they pass away. Things happen fast in the ICU, and the rooms are designed to save lives. A laptop-style computer flanks the patient's bed, positioned at standing height on a swivel stand, providing physicians with quick access to patient records, lab results, and a database of medical information.

Inside a glass cubicle at the front of the rooms, the nurse's station affords constant visual monitoring of patients; by extension, this reduces privacy to nil. ICU nurses are specially trained in critical care, and they are generally assigned only one or two patients at a time. These lifesavers represent the top professionals in their field, the very best at what they do. We also found, shortly into Jordan's stay, that many are immensely compassionate and are as deeply committed to a patient's emotional well-being as to their physical recovery.

While we waited for his results, Jordan and I became acquainted with the hospital staff. Jordan's case was attracting a miniature army. His primary physician, Dr. Richard Maziarz, a Harvard-trained hematologist and oncologist, instantly struck me as a competent, intuitive, and personable physician. A pod of doctors and medical students seemed to shadow him everywhere he went, tapping furious notes into computer tablets or scribbling away on yellow legal pads.

The next doctor to check in was the general physician in charge of the ICU, and after him, we met an infection specialist whose main function was to ensure Jordan didn't die from any secondary diseases, which often result from depressed immune functioning. This doctor was also being tailed by several other doctors, who appeared to be both in training as well as assisting with Jordan's care.

Over the coming days we also met with social workers, admissions personnel, certified nursing assistants, dietitians, physical therapists, clergy, and many others.

One of the things I picked up on right away was that none of these people were saying the sorts of things you would expect them to say in this type of situation. I mean, in movies and TV shows, the actors who play doctors always say things like, "Don't worry, kid, you're going to be all right. I've never lost a patient, and I'm not about to start now..." There was none of that. There weren't even mild reassurances. The pace of the staff was rapid. The mood was serious and leaned toward somber. The nurses provided virtually continuous care and observation. They all acted as if Jordan was in serious trouble, not unlike the ICU doctor who had first examined Jordan in the hospital back home in Bend.

This is when I paused to give Jordan my "with love, all things can be healed" speech. It was a spontaneous response, fully unplanned and unrehearsed, but as it turned out, the timing could not have been better. Within another hour, Jordan's MRI results came back, and Dr. Maziarz showed us the images. Both of Jordan's lungs were strangled with tumors. The damn things were everywhere.

CHAPTER FOURTEEN

The Power of Prayer and Affirmations

I have to admit, there was a time in my life when I didn't view prayer as being particularly important. Along the spiritual journey, the disciple eventually comes to a fork in the road where he or she begins to sense an intimate, and quite direct, connection with Source, at which point "prayer," in the traditional sense, becomes unnecessary. You start to realize that the universe already knows what you need before you even ask for it because you are one with the Source of all things; therefore, if you become aware of a need, so has God. You may also simultaneously come to understand that you often do not know what is in your own best interests anyway. As it turns out, human beings have a tendency to want precisely the things that are bound to hamper their own awakening. Likewise, some events you may judge to be "bad" turn out to be blessings in the long run. As students begin to realize this, they will naturally cease trying to control the direction and circumstances of their life at every twisting of the road. They become travelers into the present moment, their guiding rule to let life lead the way and unfold according to a higher order.

All this is true. However, there is a deeper lesson relating to prayer. From a human perspective, prayer and affirmation, its close cousin, are indeed helpful, and in this context, I consider prayer and affirmation to be essentially the same for all practical purposes. What I eventually learned is that, while Source may be aware of our needs, this does not mean that *we* are open to receiving Divine help. As a matter of fact, people are notoriously, stubbornly closed off from Source, and as has been emphasized, God cannot force anything upon you. I have gradually become convinced that if we could just solve the problem of feeling disconnected from Source, all the rest of our troubles would be healed, in which case there would, indeed, be no need for prayer.

For now, however, this is a need, and a great need at that. What we need is a bridge, a tool, a system of leverage, to help us become open to receiving the gifts of Source, and this is precisely what prayer is in its highest form. It helps *us* open up to receiving Divine intervention on our behalf. This sort of prayer does not ask for worldly possessions or experiences, but for awakening to Source's presence within us, which provides whatever we may need and heals whatever may be broken or amiss in our lives. Essentially, once the connection to Source is opened, everything else falls into place.

For this reason, the following prayers stick to requests for union, spiritual experience, and the healing that comes from these states. They do not ask for anything specific. Rather, by letting go of the notion that we need anything at all beyond connecting with Source, they recognize that our one true need is awakening.

The Power of Prayer

The first thing to understand about prayer is, it *works*. This may be a challenging notion to accept for those, like me, who have grown up immersed in the wonders of the scientific revelations of the late-twentieth and early-twenty-first centuries. Scientific studies that have examined prayer's efficacy have produced mixed findings, only adding to the confusion. In any case, my purpose is not to "prove" that prayer heals, but simply to share what I've learned. In that spirit, a couple of points about prayer stand out to me. First of all, if you believe that prayer will work, it will be more likely to work for *you*; second, if you believe prayer will not work, it will be less likely to work for *you*. Once again, we come back to this book's central point, which has surrounded all of our teachings — it is the *mind* that is the ultimate determiner of our experience.

Further, I've found that the most effective types of prayers are most often those that ask for connection, not specific results. They embody the spirit of the message, "Thy will be done," as opposed to "I want this" or "I need that." This is true even when the needs being sought are things or circumstances that Source would certainly satisfy given the requisite willingness on the re- questor's part, such as healing or the abatement of symptoms or suffering.

This does not mean, however, that Source intentionally ig- nores pleas for *specific* assistance as a punishment. I have learned through much hard-won experience that Source doesn't turn away from us. The limitations that occur with prayers tainted by ego goals relate to the fact that *we* ourselves — in our heart — view such prayers as impure. Because of this we may refuse to accept the Divine aid that could assist us with all our needs. Once again, Source cannot thrust gifts upon us when we are closed off, no matter how badly we may be in need of them. We must wel- come the help fully, on *all* levels, and if we believe that our asking is impure, we simply will not accept Source's answer. With this in mind, there are just a couple of points to remember in regards to prayer:

- Whatever your circumstances, try to keep your focus pure. Seek first and foremost only to connect with Source. Do not ask or demand anything beyond the simple requests outlined in the following prayers. If only for a moment, release all that you believe you need and open up to Source's presence. The journey is not far, since you are a part of Source. The transition into spiritual awareness involves only one tiny shift.
- When you do pray for something specific, don't let yourself feel guilty about it. Guilt will only further close you off from Source. It isn't a "sin" to ask for specific help; it's merely limiting. By doing so, you also presume to know what is best. It is better to let Spirit decide what you need because Spirit's viewpoint is omniscient and is therefore capable of understanding everyone's needs — past, present, and future.

The Art of Prayer

The following guidelines for prayer are merely suggestions, as are the specific prayers and affirmations that follow. Prayer is really an intuitive, often spontaneous, activity, and as such it is best to let Source guide you. With that said, there are a few points that bear considering. Use only one prayer per session, and set aside about ten minutes to work with it. Just as with meditation, it is helpful to find a quiet space in which to pray. Or you may wish to invite others to join you. Group prayer can be particularly powerful.

1. Begin by getting relaxed and settled, as you would during meditation. If you prefer, rather than sit, you may assume a more formal, kneeling prayer position, with your palms together at the level of your chin. The position of your body is not what's important; the quality of your focus and the openness of your heart are.
2. After you are relaxed, spend a few minutes repeating the word "peace" during every out-breath until you feel quieted

and you sense, however faintly, a connection with the peaceful space within.

3. Next, recite one of the prayers or affirmations listed below, speaking very slowly and with deep thoughtfulness. If you wish, open your eyes and read directly from the page. There is no need to say or memorize these prayers word for word. Remember, Source understands your needs already. Prayer is meant to help *you* open up to Source. Repeat the prayer several times out loud. Listen to the sound of the words, the rhythm and flow of the sentences, and consider their meaning. Take your time and feel the weight — or the *essence* — of the words. Sense the power that lies behind them; *God is behind them*. Let the words act as a bridge between your awareness and the mind of Source. You are trying to get in touch with God. This is the most sacred practice a human being is capable of.

4. After you have recited the prayer aloud a few times, be silent for several minutes, eyes closed, reaching into the quiet deep within, reaching into inner space. Think of the prayer silently in your mind several more times, again allowing the words to penetrate your consciousness.

5. Finish by sitting quietly for a few more minutes, meditating on the feeling of your breath entering your lungs and dispersing Source energy throughout your body.

Love Heals

Love heals.
I am not my body.
Love heals.
I am not my thoughts.
Love heals.
I am Spirit, only Spirit.

Love heals.
And Spirit is love.
Love heals.
I am Love, only Love.
Love heals.
Therefore I am healed.

May I Be Well

May I be well.
May my wellness bring me peace.
May my peace bring me joy.
May my joy bring me strength.
May my strength bring me health.
May I be well.

I Am Spirit

I am Spirit,
And Spirit is light.
Therefore so am I.
I am Spirit,
And Spirit is Life.
Therefore so am I.
I am Spirit,
And Spirit is love.
Therefore so am I.
I am Spirit,
And Spirit is well.
Therefore so am I.
I am Spirit.

Prayer for Awakening

Great Spirit,
Let me realize

I am core Self,
United with all Life,
And awake within You.
Great Spirit,
Let me know
I am core Self,
United with all Life,
And awake within You.
Today I choose to awaken.
Today I choose perfect peace.
Today I choose to see,
I live, I move, I breathe,
In the sacred heart of You.
Today I choose to rest,
Still, at peace, and eternally safe.
In the sacred heart of You.
Today I choose to lose my self,
To find my Self,
Awake, alive, and at peace,
In the heart of You.

Affirmation for Balance

Body, mind, Spirit,
All are one.
Spirit is healing,
Mind is calm,
Body is strong.
Body, mind, Spirit,
All are one.
All are well.
All are in balance.

What Am I?

What am I?
I am not my body.
What am I?
I am not my thoughts.
What am I?
I am not my personality.
What am I?
I am not my career.
What am I?
I am not my likes and dislikes.
What am I?
I am not my relationships.
What am I?
I am not my limitations.
What am I?
I am not my ego.
What am I?
I am not my body.
What am I?
I am Peace.
I am Light.
I am Love.
I am Life.
I am the presence that asks, *what am I?*

CHAPTER FIFTEEN

"You Mean I'm Not Going to Make It?"

I had only been this close to someone who was actively dying one other time. In July 2004, my mother rapidly deteriorated after a twenty-five-year battle with rheumatoid arthritis, an auto-immune disease that causes the immune system to attack the body it is designed to defend. This type of arthritis is not to be confused with osteoarthritis, which involves a mechanical deterioration of the joints due to time and use. Rheumatoid arthritis is a serious illness that afflicts millions of people worldwide, and it not only assaults the joints of the body — bending fingers into ghastly protuberances and crumpling hands and feet until they are barely recognizable — it can also attack a person's vital organs, including the heart.

My mom had grown progressively weaker over the years, until eventually she could no longer stand on her own without collapsing to the ground. This left her bedridden during the en-tire last two years of her life — a heart-wrenching situation that shocked our family and left us feeling both hopeless and helpless. With her medical situation growing more complicated with every passing month, she was ultimately admitted to a nursing facility. There was simply no way for us to care for her on our own without putting her life at risk.

We all hoped my mom would get better, at least well enough to come live with me and my family, which was the plan. Sadly, she never recovered, and toward the end we all began to realize that she would be stuck in a nursing home for the rest of her life. She was only sixty-seven years old.

This would be a devastating realization under any circumstances, but it was doubly brutal in my mom's case because she remained relatively lucid. Many nursing home residents suffer from dementia, and they may not be fully aware of their situation and environment. In my mom's case, this was not so, and despite the fact that the nursing home staff mostly consisted of superb, kind, and caring people, it was still a dreadful place to live. Much of the time she was left all alone in her tiny room, where she spent her days watching television to pass the time. I visited her regularly, at first spending several hours every day sitting at her bedside, but over the course of her final year, my visits tapered to only an hour a day. I stuck to this commitment religiously, but it became harder for me to bear as time dragged on.

At that time, I had no idea what I was dealing with on a psychological level, but I now realize that I had withdrawn into an emotional cocoon. I have come to understand that this is actually a normal reaction that serves an important function in these situations. This psychological protective mechanism is not all that different from the hard shell a turtle retreats into when it feels threatened. To be totally honest, I'm embarrassed to admit that over the last year of her life even spending that one hour a day visiting with her felt like an awful chore, but it is true nevertheless. From the moment I walked through her door, my mind was already fixated on getting the hell out of there. As a result,

I usually passed my one hour with her without even truly being present at all.

Dealing with illness and watching a loved one struggle helplessly can be an emotionally brutal assault. If you are close to a patient and dealing with such feelings, rest assured that this is a common reaction. You are not alone. Based on my own experience, however, I urge you to make every effort, no matter how difficult, to be present and available for your loved one as much as possible. Your presence and connection is powerful medicine, and it may serve an important role even for those patients who, like my mom, do not survive their illness.

Death is a surreal process. It may sound strange, but nobody actually ever expects anyone to die, even during the final moments of life. It's as if death is inconceivable to the living. Even after someone has passed away, it is hard to believe they're gone. It feels more like a bad dream than a reality. I believe the reason for this is that some deep, mystically aware part of us knows that death is not real. We realize, despite the evidence our eyes transmit, that it is impossible for life to really end. Life is energy; it may change in form, but it can never be depleted.

A Course in Miracles teaches that death, like sickness, is a choice. It is a decision made by the individual, not something that occurs due to random chance or fate. I have seen no greater proof of this than in the cases of my mom and Jordan, though in the end Jordan's choice was the opposite of my mother's. I remember taking my mom to a doctor's appointment one day shortly before she passed away. She was an emotional wreck that day. Just a week before, her roommate at the nursing home suddenly died. Though my mom had moved from a private room to a shared room only a few months before, she was a highly social person, and she had gotten to know this lady quite well in a short time.

Apparently, the nursing home's air conditioner went out

during a brutal heat wave the week before, and her roommate died from hyperthermia, which is essentially overheating. This is actually a common cause of death among the elderly and infirm. Heat waves kill people every year, all over the world.

Mom was devastated by her roommate's death, and she was doubly traumatized having to witness her friend's body being wheeled out of their room with a sheet pulled across her face. She finally broke down over the incident, bursting into tears while we were visiting with her doctor for a routine checkup. "I just don't know how you stand watching people die all the time," she said to her doctor, dabbing at her tear-streaked face with a crumpled tissue.

This particular physician was not known for his comforting bedside manner. Just the opposite; he tended to be abrasive and cold. Mom did not like him on a personal level, but, as fate would have it, she ended up stuck with him. On this occasion, though, her doctor paused and became deeply thoughtful before responding. He then said something that surprised me: "I see a lot of suffering, Frances, and there are times when there is just nothing more I can do to help. That is the most painful part of my job. Sometimes death is easier."

The instant he finished speaking, the whole world seemed to fall utterly silent and still. It was as if the air had been sucked from the room, and someone hit the Cosmic pause button on the temporal progression, allowing a tiny breath of eternity to infuse the space. In the same moment, I saw my mom's face change. The shift was barely perceptible, and I'm sure the doctor did not notice it, but it was something I registered clearly with an instinct I cannot quite find the words to describe. What I can tell you is that she was silent for a time, her eyes lit up with a bead of light, and a measure of her sadness seemed to evaporate.

She had made her decision then, and I knew it, somehow. Mom had decided to leave the world...

Just weeks later she was admitted to the hospital with a serious bladder infection that proved untreatable with antibiotics, and from there, things unfolded in a blur. She soon became delirious and withdrawn as the infection infested her body, and it gradually became clear she had entered an unexpected downward spiral. It wasn't long before she was transferred to a hospice and put on "comfort care," which means she would be provided whatever care and medications were needed to ensure that she was as comfortable as possible, but no attempts would be made to keep her alive.

On July 10, 2004, a mere twenty-four hours after being checked into the hospice, Mother quietly left her body while surrounded by my sisters, my ex-wife, and me — all the people who loved her most — while we held her crippled hands and shared stories about our lives together and about our love for her and each other.

I was with Jordan, too, when he made his own decision between life and death. Just as I had registered my mom's choice on some primal, indefinable level, so too did I fully recognize Jordan's decision as it flashed across his face and lit, for the briefest of moments, his eyes with life.

After the MRI results came back and revealed that the cancer had infiltrated Jordan's lungs — as well as his liver — nothing really sunk in immediately. Dr. Maziarz decided to administer a chemo drug that was a combination of a medication Jordan had already received mixed with one he hadn't yet had, in the hopes that it would stave off the cancer's progress at least long enough for Jordan's family to get to Portland, so they could explore options and make decisions.

In that immediate moment, though, they needed someone who was legally capable of making decisions for Jordan should he become unable to speak for himself, which was a real probability. Jordan asked me to do it, and I agreed without hesitation, although I knew it was a terrifying responsibility. I had also been placed in charge with a similar legal responsibility when my mom's condition became critical and she could no longer communicate her desires. I had in fact made the final decision to have her transferred from the hospital to hospice care, which led to her death within a day. Though the choice was made after much deliberation and consultation with my family and my mom's doctors, it was still an unbearably painful decision to make. I resolutely *did not* want to have to decide this for Jordan. Still, I knew immediately that it was a responsibility I could not refuse. Within a few hours, Jordan and I had signed the necessary legal paperwork, giving me his power of attorney.

By this point, though no one said it directly in plain words, Jordan's doctors were suggesting that he was probably going to die as a result of this latest infiltration of the cancer into his lungs. The most recent MRI images showed that the cancer had aggressively asserted itself in a truly alarming manner. The invasion of the cancer appeared to be a total takeover.

What the doctors *did* make clear was that since chemotherapy had already failed three times (four times if you counted the targeted therapy Jordan had received), there was little hope that anything could be done to stop this latest incursion. Cancer has a way of learning to subvert chemical treatments, just as bacteria adapts to antibiotics, which is what happened in my mom's case. Once a particular cancer has learned to get around a particular drug, that drug becomes useless.

Jordan's doctors delicately tried to help Jordan understand his situation, but at first he didn't seem to comprehend what they were suggesting. At eighteen, Jordan's innocence and trust was such that when one of his doctors asked him if he was scared to be in the ICU, he replied that he was excited to be there because "now maybe someone will do something about this." When I interviewed Jordan for this book, he admitted that he *never* expected to die. He always assumed, no matter how bad things got, that some cure would be found. In the end it may have been his absolute trust that ultimately saved him. Certainly, it played a leading role. However, at the time, and knowing full well the kind of trouble he was in, it was a heartbreaking thing to hear him voice.

Eventually the physician in charge of the ICU privately asked me if Jordan understood his situation, and I confessed that I did not think so. Later that day, that same doctor, Jordan's primary nurse, and a man whom I took to be a social worker entered Jordan's room and flanked his bedside. Apparently, it was time for "the talk."

I don't remember exactly what was said, but the fact that Jordan was dying was made clear.

"Do you understand what we're trying to tell you, Jordan?" the doctor asked.

Just then, tears came into Jordan's eyes. "You mean I'm not going to make it?"

I tried to say something, but I found I could not speak. Instead, I rested my hand on Jordan's leg and fell into silence, strangled by grief. The social worker touched Jordan's arm, and the doctor, on the other side of the bed, took Jordan's hand in his own. Everyone fell silent, and we all spontaneously closed our eyes for a few moments as time seemed to slow and pause, just as it had in my mom's case.

Moments later, the nurse who was most often caring for Jordan in the ICU came over and sat down on his bed. She then laid her entire upper body across Jordan's chest and embraced him, looking him directly in the face, only inches away. "Nobody's giving up on you," she said with a combination of sorrow and strength.

I glanced at Jordan just then and caught sight of a spark of raw determination that ignited in his eyes. It was a look remarkably similar to the one I had noted in my mom's eyes that day at her doctor's appointment years before. It was the look of a soul making an irrevocable decision. Only in this case what I saw reflected there was the decision to live.

CHAPTER SIXTEEN

Laying Hands, Holding Presence, and Unity

*I*t is my opinion that healing occurs in ways no human being can fully comprehend. While physical treatments are often involved, true healing is triggered through mysterious mechanisms known only to Source. I make no claims to understanding the process myself, at least not in its entirety. Fortunately for us, understanding the healing process from an ego level is not necessary in order for it to occur. What we do need to learn, however, are the rules that make it possible to open the doorway that leads to the *experience* that heals. The means may remain a mystery, yet this does not matter when the ego falls away and the healing dimension is at last entered.

Some of the things that may help trigger healing have surprised me. In the previous chapter on prayer, for instance, I mentioned that at one point along my spiritual journey I didn't consider prayer to be of much use, until I later realized that prayer can indeed stimulate healing in much the same way meditation can — not by asking for special favors, but by awakening the patient. Another trigger for healing that surprised me, but which

I've seen through my own direct experience (which is the most convincing way of learning), is what is sometimes referred to as "laying hands." This method of healing could also be called "healing touch."

The healing nature of touch stems from the power that is awakened when two or more human souls connect. This process actually has nothing to do with the body at all, and touch itself is not necessary in order to provoke a healing response in the patient. This is true because bodies only *seem* to separate us from each other. In Heaven, our native Homeland, there are no bodies to interpose barriers between us. There is only an endless dancing unity of Life, which is ever-expanding and creating. Therefore, any appearance of separation must be an illusion. Yet in this world the *apparent* reality of separation is thoroughly convincing. Most people never even pause to seriously question it. They go through their lives from birth to death believing they are the body their eyes behold and their hands can feel, but nothing more. From this perspective they seem to be an island unto their own, cut off from the rest of life and Source as well. This fixation on the physical makes it difficult for them to feel *any* sense of connection to another person without touch playing a part. Thus the contact point between two bodies can serve as a type of perceptual bridge through which the sense of division is temporarily dissolved and the reality of unity can be experienced.

In other words, you do not need physical contact in order to connect with others, but some people *believe* they do.

Regardless of how it is achieved, when human beings lose their sense of separate identities and unite in the awareness of their oneness, the power of God, which sleeps within all of us, is awakened. This joining is so powerful that through it *anything* becomes possible.

These moments, like all authentic healing moments, typically occur spontaneously. When Jordan's doctor, the social worker, and I all laid our hands on Jordan's body, it wasn't something any of us intended to do. At least I do not believe the others acted with conscious thought. I know I certainly did not, and it felt thoroughly unplanned on everyone's part. It seemed like in that moment, we all shared in one wish — *that this boy should heal and not die.* His disease, and the situation in general, felt like such a primitive violation of life and innocence, it was nearly unbearable, and equally unbelievable.

The moment we touched him, I felt myself transported above the level of my body, and when I closed my eyes, it seemed as if the world vanished and I found myself floating in a sea of light. I am not sure what the others experienced just then. It is quite possible their experience was more mundane. Since I am accustomed to entering such states, I recognized what was occurring right away, and allowed myself to go deeply into it. In the end it doesn't matter whether they realized anything out of the ordinary was happening or not. The full healing power of our union together was released nevertheless, and based on Jordan's response, it evidently went to work immediately.

Again, none of us tried to make this happen. What we *did* do was join in one common goal, which was the wish for Jordan to live. Such goals, which are resolutely focused on an objective with no hesitance or qualifications attached whatsoever, transcend mere wishing and rise into the realm of *willing*. In that moment, each of us in our own way *willed* Jordan to live.

As I've described, afterward the nurse who was also in the room came over and embraced Jordan in a powerful moment of healing touch, adding her own energy to the situation. On an interesting side note, the fact that her contact with Jordan occurred apart from the rest of us, separated by perhaps twenty or thirty seconds, did not appear to matter in the least. It is not only the sense of space and physical boundaries that presents an illusion of separation; time cannot divide us either. What is one in Truth has always been one. Therefore, in Reality you are equally united with those who lived a thousand years ago, as well as the billions who are yet to be born.

Although it may not be necessary to understand the mechanics through which touch heals, theoretical comprehension can still be helpful for those wanting to specifically induce a healing. As noted, laying of hands often occurs without a person's conscious intent. In the moment when I reached out and placed my hand on Jordan, I was not specifically trying to induce healing. I had let go of all personal purpose and was acting from present-moment awareness.

Yet it is possible to consciously trigger the experience of the healing dimension using touch. Like all forms of healing, it can't be forced, but if a patient is open to the possibility even for one instant, a healer may intentionally, consciously, unite with that person. This can be done in order to spark physical healing, but it can aid the healing process of situations, negative psychological states, and relationships as well. Years ago I intentionally induced healing touch to repair my relationship with Kirsten. At the time we were experiencing some serious struggles together, which I did not know how to repair. Eventually I reached a point where I suspected the relationship would end. There seemed to be no possible way to fix the things that were broken between us.

Then, one night while lying in bed next to her just before sleep, I let go of my sense of pride and ego and the drive to be right. She was lying on her side, and I snuggled close to her and pressed my body against hers. Placing my attention at the spot where her body and mine met, I used the sense of physical connection as a sort of mindfulness focus, letting it draw me into the here and now. I then intentionally allowed the sense of a boundary between us to dissolve, and I tried to feel as if there was nothing separating us — which in truth there wasn't and isn't. In this case, my intent to "try to feel no boundary" triggered a genuine experience of union.

Such states are actually easy to recognize once you become familiar with them. When they occur, you may feel as if your body has suddenly become remarkably subtle and light. Some people describe it as a sense of numbness, though the body is not actually numb; you've merely allowed your consciousness to shift beyond it. You may even feel as if your body has disappeared. During this state the important point of focus is the sensation of unity with the person sharing this sacred space with you, which is, in the grandest sense, a brief vision of the state that precedes full revelation — or so-called God realization. The experience of unity is like a middle ground that bridges earth and Heaven.

Interestingly, though Kirsten was not attempting to make anything out-of-the-ordinary happen, and she was not a conscious spiritual student at that time, she nevertheless experienced the union, too, and it felt the same to her as it did to me.

A related technique, which I refer to as "holding presence," can be thought of as an advanced form of laying hands that does not require physical touch. Because the body does not actually separate us from one another, the physical part of the method is actually unnecessary. The steadfast, fixed belief that we must be in physical contact in order to experience a state of union with another person is not true. Advanced healers who understand this point can initiate the awareness of unity through their presence alone.

Much of my time with Jordan, whether in the hospital or out of it, was spent holding only one awareness in mind — the clear-cut understanding of my absolute and indivisible link with him. I tried not only to remember this connection intellectually but to experience it directly, for herein lies the real healing power of this technique. Believing something is true can open you to the experience of it, but it is only the experience itself that carries the power to heal. I knew that if I was able to hold the awareness of our unity firmly in mind, Jordan's awareness of unity would also be kindled, if only subconsciously.

To be clear, a healer doesn't *cause* healing; the healer's presence, centered on unity, merely reminds the patient of the presence of the healing dimension, so that the patient is gently encouraged toward healing without fear. This can occur because the patient's and the healer's minds are indeed one already, so that what one feels feeds directly into the other's mental-emotional body.

Much of Jordan's healing occurred silently in the unseen world that surrounds and unites us with one another and with our Source. This is also why no particular words are necessary in order for a healing to be triggered, nor any special procedures or rituals of any sort. You don't need to light candles, burn sage, or chant mantras under a full moon — though, to reiterate, these things can indeed be helpful if a patient *believes* they possess some healing capacity of their own. Such is the power of belief. The same could be said of physical healing procedures, doctors, and all forms of medication as well.

Remember, the goal is only to help the patient reach the healing dimension, however he or she attains that connection. Therefore, whatever healing methods feel most natural and appealing, and that align most closely with the patient's belief system, are probably the ones that should be attempted first. The saying "go with the flow" is wise advice in many situations, and most especially when it comes to the delicate process of recovery. Why fight against beliefs and a thought system that is already in place when it can be harnessed to lead the patient to true healing?

Laying Hands and Healing Touch

Once again, healing touch often occurs spontaneously without any conscious intent, but just as with entering the healing dimension, you can practice the procedure and by doing so potentially invoke the experience. Even if you do not have a full healing experience from this exercise, even casual human contact is charged with healing potential.

1. Begin by adopting a seated or lying position next to the patient.

2. Quiet your thoughts as much as possible before starting. Some people like to begin by reciting prayers or affirmations, either spoken aloud or internally; others prefer to remain silent. Do whichever feels most natural. As always, the critical preparation is aligning with the now.

3. When you are ready, lay one or both of your hands somewhere along the patient's body in a nonsexual location. It is easy for touch to be interpreted sexually. If this perception does occur to either party, simply allow the feeling to pass and don't cling to it. It is natural enough, and you should not feel ashamed or embarrassed by the reaction. If several people are participating, the group should also place their hands on the patient at about the same time, though perfect synchronicity is not necessary. In close relationships, or for those who are comfortable, the touch can include a full embrace or hug,

from the front or aligned — body-to-body — from behind, either while lying down or sitting up.

4. Next, focus your attention at the point of contact between your bodies. Let your attention be drawn to the sense of physical contact. Then gradually feel as if the boundaries between your bodies are dissolving, as if there is no barrier there at all. Imagine that you are not two bodies, closed off from each other by physical borders, but one soul directly joined and existing in a single body that itself has no firm boundary, but which extends without limit into infinity.

5. To whatever degree you can, attempt to experience this directly and go deeply into it. Feel as if the two of you exist together, floating, in a warm cocoon of safety filled with healing light. Let the sensation of unity fully envelop you. Most of all focus on deep relaxation.

6. Spend a few minutes, or as long as you and the patient are comfortable, dwelling in this space. When you are done, open your eyes and sit together quietly.

Holding Presence

This technique is ideally performed while in the same room with the patient, but it can be done at any distance, since neither time nor space actually separates the patient from the healer. Still, close physical proximity may help solidify the experience and so facilitate focus.

1. Ideally you should perform this from a seated position with your eyes closed, but advanced healers can do it with eyes open while either standing or sitting.

2. Get relaxed and draw your awareness to the present. Once again, if it helps, focus your attention on the sensation of air entering and exiting your body.

3. For advanced healers, steps three and four may be replaced by a simple awareness of the unity that exists between you and the patient. However, the following visual exercise may help you make a connection with the patient: Summon an image of the patient in your mind. See the person as clearly as possible in your imagination. Then imagine the person's body being gradually enveloped in a healing golden light, until it vanishes in the glow.

4. Now see your own body enveloped in an identical light, then imagine the light expanding toward the patient until it connects the two of you, merging you both into one sphere of light.

5. Meditate on the feeling of unity with the patient as long as you feel comfortable, and, as always, be sure to sit quietly for at least a few minutes afterward, holding the sense of peace and unity in your awareness.

CHAPTER SEVENTEEN

The Mystery of the Melting Tumors

The driving theory behind spiritual healing is that, while healing itself does not occur through medications, physical treatments, or healers per se — but through the patient's own desire to heal — once the patient has chosen recovery, medications, treatments, and healers may all begin working, even if they were previously ineffectual. In this sense they are not the *cause* of healing, but a tool to bring the cause, which is the patient's own will and desire, into material being. With the decision to heal in place, the patient is bound to discover some treatment that will work. When the patient is ready, the right medication will be found; the perfect healer will show up at the perfect moment; a medication that had not worked before will suddenly begin working; or the patient may spontaneously recover.

Certainly, when Dr. Maziarz started Jordan on yet another course of chemotherapy, none of us, including Jordan's doctors, expected it to accomplish much. Yet something *had* to be done. They couldn't just do nothing and let the cancer consume him without some attempt at a fight.

After "the talk" with the ICU doctor, I immediately contacted Kirsten, my daughter Brittany, and other close family members in order to let them know what was happening. I urged everyone to find a way to come to Portland as quickly as possible. Likewise, Jordan contacted his family in the hopes that they, too, would come be with him. Jordan had mixed emotions about having his mom there. On the one hand, of course, he *wanted* her support; on the other, he didn't want any more conflict, and due to her own unhealed wounds, she was not handling Jordan's illness well. However, her presence was important to Jordan, and he set aside any uncertainty and relayed to her exactly what the doctor had said.

This was the most painful moment in the journey. Not only was Jordan dying, but things were progressing rapidly. We really had no idea how long the cancer could be held off, and Jordan was already consuming a large amount of bottled oxygen, which was a dire sign. To say that everyone was devastated by the news would be an understatement. *Shattered* would be a better description. Brittany, my older daughter Ashley, and their mom immediately made arrangements for the trip to Portland. They anticipated arriving within the next two or three days. At this point they expected that it would be to say good-bye.

Meanwhile, the ICU nurse and I also connected with Jordan's school. As timing would have it, Jordan was supposed to be graduating from high school in just a few days. He had worked hard for the achievement, overcoming a variety of obstacles, and it seemed like a cheat for him not to graduate, despite his current circumstances. The problem was, he still had one final assignment that needed completion before he could graduate, and it was a *mandatory* project, required by Oregon state law. The world's rules, it seemed, could not be broken, even for death!

However, with some prying, we discovered that they could be bent just a little...

After consulting with his teachers and the school's adminis-
tration, it was deemed Jordan could turn in a simplified version of
the final project, which he rapidly completed with just a little help.
Assuming he lived long enough, Jordan would graduate after all.
Death would not intervene. In a way this was a bittersweet victory, being both an accomplishment and at the same time a testament to the unfairness of the moment. That such a young, bright
boy was about to be ripped away from life and all those who loved
him when his journey was only just beginning aroused an excru-
ciating sense of injustice in everyone. Yet there was nothing to
be done. Jordan would graduate in a hospital room hundreds of
miles away from home, symbolically completing his metamorphosis from childhood into adulthood. How long he would live as
an adult beyond this moment was impossible to tell. All we knew
for certain was *un*certainty.

That afternoon one of Jordan's buddies arrived from Bend,
pretending to be Jordan's stepbrother. Apparently, he had been
wrongly informed that the ICU would only allow family to visit,
so he decided to fib his way in. In any case, the visit was a welcome relief. It allowed me to take a break from my bedside vigil
and get away to clear my thoughts.

While in Portland I was staying with a close friend of mine
who lived in the area. That day when I returned to her house, I
realized how traumatized, helpless, and drained I was by Jordan's
situation. You remember that waterfall analogy? This was the
moment when the falls were looming and hopelessness consumed
me. I desperately needed support, but I felt that I couldn't unbur-
den myself on my friend. The truth is, her husband had committed suicide just the year before (which I mentioned in chapter 1),

and the wound was still fresh for her. Death was a painful subject, and I did not want to cause her any unnecessary duress.

Instead, I turned to my spiritual Teacher. Early that evening I isolated myself in my friend's guest room and opened *A Course in Miracles*. I voraciously read one random selection after the next, meditating on each of the passages in a desperate attempt to stabilize my emotional state. The first section the book opened to was one I had not read in years, titled "Holy Week." In part, it says, "This is Palm Sunday, the celebration of the victory and the acceptance of truth.... Easter is a sign of peace, not pain.... This week we celebrate life, not death."

For those unfamiliar with this great spiritual teaching, *A Course in Miracles* has a bizarre propensity for syncing up with whatever a student happens to be going through at any given time and providing brilliant guidance. As it turned out, I continually encountered this particular section of the *Course* during this week with Jordan. The words I was reading were clear enough, and by this time in my life I had come to deeply trust the *Course*'s guidance, but the present situation was beyond anything I'd had to deal with since my mom's death. Thus, despite my Teacher's reassuring message, I remained steadfastly *un*-reassured.

Upon trying to meditate that evening I found that my mind was overrun by fear thoughts and wild projections into the future, and I eventually realized I had allowed myself to become actually *frantic*.

What was I to do? How could I stop this?! How was I to comfort my daughter? Jordan was truly dying. It was hard to accept, almost unbelievable, and yet it was true. A part of me felt betrayed by God. I did not then, nor do I now, believe in major coincidences. Yet I could not wrap my head around the notion that I was simply present in this situation to comfort this kid during his passage from his earthly existence, which is what it was seeming like. The whole time Jordan had been ill, I had always assumed I was there to help him heal. Perhaps I had been wrong. Not only was Jordan going to die, which was an unthinkable disaster, but I also felt like a failure as a teacher, a failure as a healer, and a failure as a father due to my inability to protect my daughter from the agony she was about to face.

When I finally decided to try to get some sleep, fear thoughts ravaged me for hours, and I tossed and turned helplessly in bed. Eventually 1:30 a.m. rolled around, then 2:00, then 2:30.... Perhaps half an hour or so later I gave up trying to sleep and found myself sitting up in the darkness, meditating. I struggled with my mind, trying to quiet it, but my efforts proved utterly useless at first. I'm not sure how much time passed, but at some point I became exhausted.

And that's when it happened. Quite suddenly something gave way and I let go and shifted inward. Without my prompting, my thoughts grew utterly silent, and my body and mind fell into a deep stillness; even the physical world seemed to retreat and become enveloped in a magical bubble, as if the strange hush had settled across the whole city. I felt as if I had been lifted up and out of my body, above my fear, and far beyond the troubles of my mortal existence on earth.

What a relief!

I later realized that I had been forced into this sublime state as the result of sheer mental exhaustion. It is true that sometimes pain is precisely the thing we need in order to drive us to awaken, however uncomfortable it may be at the time.

I do not know how long I remained in that space because time in such states tends to become distinctly distorted, but the next thing I knew it was eight in the morning and I awoke feeling refreshed, albeit still anxious. I pulled myself out of bed, showered, and hurriedly ate breakfast. By the time I climbed into my car and headed for the hospital, Portland's morning traffic had thinned enough to allow for an easy commute into the city. As it turned out, I was right on schedule. When I arrived, Jordan was just returning to his room after getting another MRI. He had also had more blood drawn and sent for additional tests. His doctors wanted to see exactly what the cancer was up to.

Jordan and I spent that morning together mostly in silence. Under such tense circumstances, people don't always want to talk about their situation. Rather than attempt to vent their fears and comfort themselves through conversation, oftentimes the opposite occurs; patients and those close to them shut down in order to shield themselves from the nightmare. It's a natural enough response. I have found that most people in these circumstances need some quiet time during which the situation is left behind as much as possible, as well as periods during which it is openly discussed. Like so many things in life, balance is essential. In this case, both of us seemed to be simultaneously drawn into a similar silent reprieve.

Dr. Maziarz and his entourage entered the room a bit later in the day and immediately circled the computer at Jordan's bedside. The results from the MRI and lab tests were in. I watched as Dr. Maziarz scanned the page, then clicked on another. He scrolled down, examining the information thoughtfully. I watched his face for any sign of what was coming, attempting to read his mind, feeling more numb than anything else at this point.

Dr. Maziarz's eyes gradually widened and his face displayed clear surprise as he continued scrolling and reading, then a grin crossed his face. The other physicians who were at his side exchanged glances and could not help smiling, too. Eventually, Dr. Maziarz turned to Jordan. "How are you feeling?" he asked.

Jordan nodded. "Okay, I guess."

In fact, Jordan did look remarkably better than he had the day before.

Dr. Maziarz shook his head in astonishment. He spun the computer around and showed us an image of Jordan's chest, which had been captured just that morning. It revealed that both lobes of Jordan's lungs now appeared to be almost completely clear, whereas before they had looked like a connect-the-dots puzzle laced with cancer. It was almost too much to comprehend. The tumors had literally melted away overnight.

CHAPTER EIGHTEEN

Support Networks and Spiritual Relationships

O ne of the most important things a person can have during
any illness is dedicated, loving support. Just the sense of
care alone that is aroused when people gather together in a unified show of love makes a powerful statement. Besides offering
practical help in numerous forms, support networks also serve to
remind the patient, through their concern and presence, that the
patient is not alone.

A strong support network also benefits other members of the
patient's team by sharing the demands an illness inevitably creates, as well as seeing to the emotional needs of one another. It is
not only the sick who suffer. All of the patient's friends, family,
and acquaintances also experience stress, and for those who are
closest to the patient, the situation may well become a major life
stressor without adequate help.

Disease often creates a rift of distress that spreads outward
in an arc from the patient, like an earthquake expanding from its
epicenter. The form this distress may take is apt to vary from person to person. Certainly emotional turmoil is felt to some degree

by everyone involved, but physical suffering may occur as well. These symptoms may or may not appear to be linked to the patient's illness. When a specific disease physically "spreads" from one person to another — such as the flu — the direct passage of the illness is easy to identify. But if a patient has cancer, let's say, which is not communicable, and a relative experiences a heart attack, the common bond between the two conditions is less clear, even though they may well be indirectly linked, if nothing else, due to the stress of the situation. Of course, this is an extreme example. A patient's support team usually experiences physical symptoms that are far less severe, and possibly no more than a depression of the immune system, leading to an increase in various infections and generalized complaints.

Besides physical symptoms and emotional distress, other stressors may come into play. For example, the patient's family may suffer financial difficulties as the result of their loved one's illness. According to the journal *Health Affairs*, at least half of all bankruptcy cases list disease and the associated bills as a major contributing factor. Even when medical treatments are covered by insurance companies, this does not account for deductibles, time missed from work, as well as travel, food, and hotel expenses when visiting distant treatment centers, which is a common scenario during a serious illness.

For all these reasons and more, support teams often find that they need one another as much as the patient needs them. It is critical that those involved in caring for the patient, in any way, understand these stressors and prepare themselves to process and deal with them in a positive way. As with all our lessons, this one begins with awareness. Physical disease, unstable emotions, anxiety, and depression are all common symptoms caused by the stress of watching someone you care about suffer. This is inevitable and to some degree perhaps unavoidable. Members of the support team, therefore, must resolve not to project their own stress, fear, and uncertainty onto others who are also trying to help. This may require a conscious, determined effort to be doubly patient with the feelings of others as well as more aware of your own emotional state. One helpful approach is to use the situation, however negative it seems, as an opportunity to fortify your connections with those around you; others will be experiencing the same fears and challenges you are dealing with. As you learn to communicate in positive ways about difficult things, you may take your relationships in a new, healthier direction, leading to unexpected heights of learning, compassion, and wisdom. All situations, no matter how challenging, can be used for healing.

Healthy Relationships

Without a doubt, no component of healing is more important than healthy relationships. Our relationships are the single most important factor to living a happy, healthy life in general. Without rich, satisfying relationships, your life will always feel incomplete and impoverished, no matter how rich your worldly circumstances. In my view, relationships are more important to our happiness than money, success, education, and physical health combined. As long as we have strong relationships, we can do without any one of these things and still feel loved and, by extension, happy. However, if our relationships are lacking, no amount of money, success, or health will matter. You can have all the money in the world, attain the height of success in your career, and be the most physically fit and healthiest person on the planet, but if your relationships are a wreck, you will be too — at least on the inside, where it counts. There is no escaping what you hold within; the content of your heart and head accompanies you wherever you go.

In the end, all we really have are our connections with other people. As the old saying goes, you cannot take your money, or any possession, with you when you die. This is true of every worldly asset you will ever have. None of it belongs to you. The things of time and space forever belong to time and space. They are on loan, and that is all. Therefore they are not truly yours. The one thing you can take with you is the love you have shared with others because, as many mystics have noted, love is what we are; it is literally what our souls are made of. Therefore all the love you give and receive while in Earth School is added to your being. This may sound trite, but it is nevertheless true. I know this for a certainty because I have had the good fortune to glimpse the world that lies beyond our own on numerous occasions, and I have seen what all the mystics of history have seen. You don't have to take my word on this. You too can learn to see the nature of your soul very easily. All it requires is sustained effort, desire, and basic mind training.

This is why healthy relationships are so important. Of all the topics and methods for healing discussed in this book, striving to cultivate loving, healed relationships is without a doubt the most important. If you are able to perfect your relationships to the point where you offer only love to all the people in your life — whether they represent keystone relationships, acquaintances, or are merely strangers you happen to meet briefly only once — you will be well on your way to living a healthy life, both emotionally and physically. Developing healthy relationships may represent the ultimate human goal and, without a doubt, is one of the most challenging accomplishments we can achieve.

The problem is very few of us attain such perfection when it comes to our personal relationships. If you are like most people, perhaps you have noticed that virtually all the major stressors in your life come from dealing with other human beings — and stress and conflict feed disease like no other earthly toxin. Researchers talk a lot about the many carcinogens we are exposed to in the modern world, but none that I know of have identified the ultimate carcinogen, which is our toxic relationships with one another.

On the other hand, the ultimate healthy relationship is called a spiritual relationship, and these have a powerful, positive effect on our health. Spiritual relationships go beyond merely being "healthy." Spiritual relationships are based on awakening to the unity that connects two souls, joining them together as one.

Spiritual Relationships

It could be argued that *all* relationships are inherently spiritual because the underlying truth is that human beings are spiritual in nature. Therefore your real relationships with others do not exist between egos but between souls. Yet the spiritual relationship is one that places this awareness at the center of its identity. This relationship holds the realization of unity as its highest aim. This may not be a conscious goal at the outset of the relationship, but when it does become conscious, the relationship is bound to evolve into a powerful alliance that leads both to exhilarating heights of awareness.

All this does not necessarily mean that such relationships will be conflict free. The idea that spiritual relationships are "perfect" is a common misnomer. The spiritual relationship is really an unfolding process of purification through which forgiveness is practiced over and over. It may never be fully mastered during the course of the relationship, but every successful effort provides sweeping learning gains. This is how unity is eventually realized — through forgiveness, which is really only a process that removes elements of division between people. Yet no relationship can be considered perfect because neither participant is perfect, at least not on an earthly level. This much is a given. If they were, they would not be students of Earth School. However, the primary difference between the spiritual relationship and ego-bound relationships is that the spiritual relationship emphasizes releasing the past and forgiving mistakes, whereas destructive ego relationships are heavily engaged in maintaining grievances and reinforcing guilt; egos clash, divide, and assault, whereas spirits unite, seek to make happy, and heal.

The process of developing a strong, conscious spiritual relationship may take many years, but it does not need to. The sooner and more deeply the participants in the relationship are able to accept absolute, unconditional forgiveness and love for the other, the sooner any conflict will end.

Every spiritual relationship is unique, but all of them contain certain central, common characteristics that make them what they are. The development of these characteristics will move your relationships in the direction of healing, no matter the formal roles of those involved:

- **Spiritual relationships are supportive, not destructive.** It is fine if relationships challenge you to grow; indeed, they should. But spiritual relationships are based on mutual respect and care. Your relationships should help you feel secure, safe, and nourished — mentally, emotionally, and physically.

- **Spiritual relationships are based on unconditional love, not control.** Unconditional love means that your affection for someone is not dependant on his or her behavior or values. Your love is always present and runs so deep there is no thought of it subsiding or ending due to circumstances or what you might deem "misbehavior." This does not mean that the relationship will remain in a static form, and as noted it certainly does not mean it will be conflict free. Indeed, many spiritual relationships outwardly change as they evolve and may even seem to end. However, once the inner awareness of unity is established, the relationship becomes eternal.

Perfect love, the ideal state of love that should be shared in the ideal spiritual relationship, is like sunshine. The sun does not choose which trees, flowers, or people to shine upon. It does not shed more of its warmth on pine trees and less to aspens because it thinks pines are more worthy, beautiful, or fragrant. It simply gives of its light without judging the recipient's worth or value.

- **Spiritual relationships focus on giving, not on taking.** The more you give to your relationship, the more satisfying it will become for both of you; likewise, the more you attempt to take from the relationship, the less substance there will be for both partners to draw upon. Simply put, when you take from a relationship, you deprive it; when you give to a relationship, you enrich it. I call this the *Don't Ask, Don't Expect Principle*. As much as possible, give, don't take. Ask nothing of the other; offer everything, and you will find that somehow, to your astonishment, your relationship will give back to you all you could ever hope for and more.

- **Spiritual relationships help you discover your inherent completeness, not completeness in someone else.** One of the most common misconceptions of a healed relationship is that it pairs "soul mates." If you are looking for your "soul mate," you may end your search now. You have already found this person — you. Healthy relationships are founded on the premise that each partner is *already* complete. Neither requires someone else to make them feel whole. Spiritual relationships only become possible when both partners have accepted their completion independently of the other. Once this occurs, they then become capable of sharing their mutual fullness and satisfaction with the rest of the world as a unified being. It is not that they become one. Rather, they recognize the oneness that has always been there.

- **Spiritual relationships seek to absolve guilt, not increase it.** Anytime you find yourself trying to make another person feel guilty, you can be sure you are behaving in a way that is destructive to both you and your partner, as well as to the relationship as a whole. You cannot cause another person to feel guilty without suffering guilt yourself. This is a basic, universal cause-and-effect principle: what you focus on you feed with energy, thereby making it larger from your own perspective. Whenever you feel angry, it is a symptom of the projection of guilt. Whenever you choose to forgive, it is a sign that you are working to heal guilt. By doing so, you help purify the relationship and transform it into a spiritual alliance.

When a relationship evolves into a union based on the above characteristics, the participants enter into a spiritual association, even if they don't think of it that way. The unification of two wills into one focus — with forgiveness and unconditional love as their compass — brings both into close contact with Source energy. This is precisely where spiritual relationships derive their healing power from, and why they can even be used to heal others outside of the primary relationship.

Any relationship can become a spiritual relationship because *all* relationships contain a spiritual core. Just as you have a core Self, so too do all your worldly relationships contain a Divine, purified reflection, which is your core Self's relationship with another's core Self. You may believe that you cannot salvage some of your relationships because they are too damaged, but all you really need to decide is what you want. Do you want distrust, grievances, and pain? Or would you prefer joy, healing, and the peace that comes from a unified partnership? This is really all you are choosing between. Once you decide for peace, the means to bring your relationship in line with your goal will happen naturally with very little effort required on your part. Those relationships that are destined to end because one partner is prepared to experience a holy relationship while the other is not tend to end promptly and without a lot of drama, making way for a more appropriate partner for each person.

Therefore focus only on your own readiness, and leave the details of your newborn spiritual relationship to God.

When Key Relationships Are Damaged

The first partner in a relationship to realize the need for healing becomes responsible for acting on behalf of salvaging the bond. When you find yourself engaged in endless volleys of attack with someone you love, the main thing you need to do is be willing to cease your own attacks. You cannot force someone else to change or accept that they are wrong. *You* must be the one to challenge your own need to be defensive, to justify your own attacks, and by doing so reinforce your ego. This brings us to the primary, guiding rule for healing any relationship:

Seek only to heal yourself.

This determination represents the leading shift toward authentic healing. Next must come the natural step of turning inward in order to examine your personal motivations in the conflict, with the central goal of healing your own head and heart. Forget about what you believe your partner needs to do, how they should act, and what type of attitudinal shifts you think they must undergo in order for the relationship to be improved. The belief that others must change in order for *you* to be happy is an endless ego device for ensuring that no real change will occur. As long as you maintain such a backward belief, you will *never* find happiness and peace with another because you will never be happy and at peace with yourself. There will always *seem* to be something wrong, something that needs changing, some lack of fulfillment that will follow you through life from one disappointing circumstance to the next.

In order to end any conflict you must first become willing to relinquish your own vendetta and claim on guilt against the other. For this, true forgiveness must play a central role, which simply means that you become willing to release the past and focus only on the love that can be felt in the now. This focus will also clear your mind of any unsettled personal guilt, for by no longer seeking to reinforce guilt in your partner, you will automatically extend this same courtesy to yourself. This liberates you from the misperception that your own mistakes — whether they are hidden in unconsciousness or glaring at the forefront of your awareness — are unforgivable. This is the real beauty that sets forgiveness apart from all other worldly gifts. True forgiveness benefits both parties.

Whenever you feel lost in a relationship and begin to question its value, remember that the spiritual relationship is simple, not complex, resting only on learning to give and receive love freely — and *nothing more*. Also remember that this arrangement necessarily involves a great many lessons on forgiveness because forgiveness is what you are here to learn. It is the great lesson of Earth School.

In regards to health and healing specifically, just remember that your interactions with other people provide you with much more than mere companionship. We share love and affection with one another every day, and each exchange either provides a healing elixir for our trials and our pains or it delivers a poison that will eventually lead to our own destruction. Each bond you share with another human being represents a link that connects you to Source energy, the ultimate creative, and curative, force. If you want to heal, you need look no further than your relationships. By remembering your connection with others, you are remembering your connection with God; and by loving others, you are loving God. Could anything be more healing than that?

CHAPTER NINETEEN

A String of "Co-Incidences"

By the next day Jordan's lungs had cleared so much he was taken off supplementary oxygen. The retreat of the cancer was remarkable, and while it was certainly a victory, the battle was not yet won by any stretch of the imagination. Nobody labored under the delusion that this singular success, no matter how unexpected and noteworthy, meant that Jordan had been cured. On the contrary, we knew that this particular lymphoma had shown great propensity for adapting to chemo drugs and aggressively defeating them over short periods of time, which meant it would very likely, and perhaps more quickly than ever, overcome this treatment, too.

"We need a backup plan," I said to Dr. Maziarz.

"We agree," one of the other attending physicians inserted. "We're already working on it." She sounded excited.

Dr. Maziarz then explained that by chance some of their colleagues at OHSU were currently in the process of setting up a trial of an experimental drug called Xalkori, a targeted therapy that was designed to treat Jordan's specific form of lymphoma.

It was a remarkable coincidence. Had Jordan been at any other hospital, this possibility may never have been discovered. There was a catch, however: the drug wasn't approved to be prescribed for lymphoma yet. That's what the trial was designed to help establish. This meant that Jordan would need to be accepted as a test subject into the trial in order to legally receive the drug.

"We don't want to get our hopes up just yet because Jordan's case is complicated," Dr. Maziarz conceded, "but we're pushing to get him in."

All we could do was wait.

As this nerve-racking drama was unfolding, Brittany and her mother arrived at last, bearing much-needed support. They also brought with them one additional gift: Jordan's cap and gown for his graduation. That afternoon, Jordan donned both and we preserved the celebration with a snapshot taken on Brittany's cell phone right there in the ICU. By this point Jordan was strong enough to get out of bed on his own, and he even provided one of his heart-winning smiles to christen the moment. He may have been hundreds of miles away from his graduating classmates, but in spirit I'm certain he was more than present. By now the whole school had heard about Jordan's circumstances, and being well-liked by both his classmates and the school's staff, he was on many of their minds as they crossed the stage at Marshall High and accepted their diplomas.

Of course, given all Jordan had been through, the day felt far more significant than just a high school graduation ceremony. Jordan was still fighting for his life, but the recent upturn of events had infused us with a meager dose of hope. Although we were left hanging with terrifying uncertainties, we prayed that we were celebrating much more than Jordan's graduation from high school; we hoped we were celebrating his healing and his graduation from death to life.

The celebratory mood did not last long. Dr. Maziarz delivered the bad news later that same day. It seemed Jordan's case was simply too complex for him to be considered as a candidate for the trial. The news was crushing. Drug research of this nature depends on simple cases in part so that the results are less likely to be muddled by extenuating circumstances. In this case, researchers needed patients who had simple lymphoma. Since Jordan's disease had already attacked his lungs and liver, he was quickly ruled out.

But, Dr. Maziarz informed us, *there was one additional possibility*, and it became yet another curious, unexplainable coincidence that made us all feel as if we had just stepped outside of reality and into a fictional movie, one whose plot twists followed the whims of some unseen, deviously creative screenwriter. Though the drug in question had not been approved for the treatment of lymphoma, it *had* been approved to treat *lung cancer!* It is a rare moment that anyone can say, and truly mean, that lung cancer is a blessing. Yet in this case, in this moment, that was precisely what all of us were thinking. Had it not been for the fact that the lymphoma had infiltrated Jordan's lungs, Xalkori would have been out of the question due to legal limitations.

Dr. Maziarz went on to tell us it would still be tricky to acquire, although he did not specify why. But, he reassured us, he had "contacts," and he was going to try to call in some "favors." He would let us know as soon as he heard back.

Did I mention that patients and their families do a lot of waiting?

The mechanisms through which Xalkori works are complicated, and it is only used to treat very specific cancers that are caused by abnormal ALK genes. Essentially, the medication works by disrupting the action of these genes, thereby slowing cancer growth and reducing tumor sizes. At this point, clinical trials had shown real promise, and it was already being considered significantly more effective than traditional chemotherapies for the types of cancers it was designed to treat. However, like many powerful, anticancer drugs, Xalkori can also have dangerous side effects, including liver failure and life-threatening swelling of the lungs. Suffice it to say, while we were all excited about the possibility of Jordan receiving the drug, it presented its fair share of unique concerns as well.

We didn't get the final word that Jordan had been approved to receive Xalkori until late the next day. By this time, Jordan's brother and his mom had also arrived in Portland, as had my oldest daughter, Ashley, along with her boyfriend. They were all expecting to find Jordan actively dying and were stunned by his improved condition. That's how quickly things had changed. None of us really knew what to make of it, and we hadn't shared word of his improvement because those of us who had witnessed it were still processing it ourselves. We were unsure what it meant for his prognosis and how long his reprieve would last.

With the new arrivals, Jordan finally had a full support network in place, and the timing was perfect. Things were about to get complicated, as if they weren't already difficult enough. After Jordan got the medical okay to receive Xalkori, we then had to wait on approval from his insurance company. This became a fiasco that dragged on to the point that another day passed before we were finally cleared to order the prescription. However, this was only the first of several hurdles we ultimately faced. The next snag in the process was that, for some reason, we had to order the meds directly from the manufacturer and have them shipped to a private residence. The hospital and its physicians could have nothing to do with the process. They would neither order the meds nor receive them. Once again, the exact reason for this clandestine maneuver was never clarified, but at this point none of us was willing to ask any delicate questions.

After scrambling to figure out the best place to have the medication delivered (we eventually chose Jordan's brother's girlfriend's parents' house in Gresham, Oregon, a neighboring city) we managed to get hold of the company and — at last! — placed an order for a thirty-day supply. It was now late on a Wednesday afternoon, and the Xalkori was due to ship out the next day, overnight, via FedEx. If all went well, we would have the pills on Friday.

Suffice it to say, it was a long wait. Days had already passed since Jordan's remarkable turnaround, and all that was holding the cancer in check was the chemotherapy drug. He would continue to receive chemo until his new medication arrived, but none of us, his doctors included, trusted the chemo to hold. We had all seen this scenario too many times before. With every passing day, and in fact with every hour, we feared the treatment might fail and plunge Jordan back into a life-threatening crisis. The saying "waiting on pins and needles" doesn't begin to describe the level of tension that was aroused by the numerous delays.

When Friday dawned we anxiously awaited the call saying the pills had been safely received. The plan was for Jordan's brother and his girlfriend to wait at her parents' house and rush the pills to the hospital immediately.

Noon came and went, then 1 p.m., then 2 p.m. Still no pills... Horrible thoughts filled my mind. What was going on? Had the pills been lost? Had the company decided that for legal reasons they were going to turn Jordan down after all? Finally, I called the company. Apparently, there had been some mix up. The pills had never been shipped! It seemed that the pharmaceutical company had some mysterious, last-minute "questions" they needed answered, and for some unexplained reason they had been unable to reach anyone by phone. I was told I needed to talk to one of the company's administrators, and I was transferred directly to his private extension, whereupon I proceeded to field a battery of inquiries regarding Jordan's condition. The key question, however, that they wanted clarified was, "What are the pills going to be used to treat?"

Not sure what any of this meant, I answered honestly: "Lung cancer, but Jordan also has lymphoma...and liver cancer, too."

A few moments of silence passed, during which I literally held my breath. Then the man said, "Okay, I apologize for the mix up. We'll have those shipped out to you immediately."

"When will they arrive? Is there any way to get them to us by tomorrow?" I tried not to sound too frantic, but I doubt I did a very good job of concealing my anxiety.

"It's too late today," he said. "The soonest we can get them to you is Monday."

Monday! Are you kidding me? My heart sank. This person obviously didn't realize how dire the situation was, how important each day might be. I tried explaining to him, and he was sympathetic, but there was simply nothing that could be done. The meds were located on the East Coast; we were on the West Coast. Time and space were running an interference play that there was no way around.

The weekend that followed would be one of the longest of my life.

CHAPTER TWENTY

A Brief Guide for Friends, Family, and Healers

*B*efore Jordan became ill, I never thought of myself as a "healer" per se. Although I had studied *A Course in Miracles* for over twenty years, I had restricted my use of the principles I'd learned regarding mind-body healing to myself and those closest to me who occasionally approached me for advice. The role of healer wasn't one I consciously chose, nor even desired.

In general, I considered myself a writer and meditation teacher, but I carried no particular aspirations beyond those two roles. Part of my reluctance no doubt stemmed from my mother's struggle near the end of her life, which had left me with deep negative feelings about diseases and their treatments. I had spent too many hours in hospitals, doctor's offices, and nursing homes watching my mom suffer, and a significant part of her misery derived directly from the endless medications and treatments she had endured over the years. It wasn't only her disease that had caused her death.

Jordan's situation collided with my life most unexpectedly, and as a result of my initial latent resistance, I refused to accept the role I knew, instinctively, that I was meant to play in his journey until his situation had become very serious. In the beginning I just assumed he would be fine, that the chemotherapy would work and there would be no long-term complications, no life-or-death struggle. At least this is what I told myself. Clearly I was mistaken. Nevertheless, had it not been for the fact that Jordan's life had become intimately intertwined with my daughter's, I probably would not have gotten involved at all, at least not directly.

Sometimes, the changes we are most resistant to prove to be the most powerful, critical shifts in our destiny — the ones that really change us at a fundamental level and send us hurtling off in unexpected directions. As has been observed by many others before me, God knows our strengths better than we do, and what seems a bad thing at first may unexpectedly transform into a good thing. This was certainly true in regard to the journey I undertook with Jordan Young.

I still do not really consider myself a healer, at least not any more than any of us are. I have come to learn that we are all healers in some respect, because the chief purpose of the world *is* healing. Only healers and those in need of healing inhabit Earth School, for the world is ultimately a hospital for suffering souls. The illness we suffer from is the state of illusory separation from Life, and its primary symptoms are fear states and disease. Part of the design of this hospital, however, is that as the sick are healed, they too become a part of the world's healing — a part of the solution. In a sense, we all become therapists, nurses, and doctors as we begin our ultimate healing journey into the remembrance of who we really are and where our true Home abides.

Therefore this section is meant for you, Dear Reader, whoever you are and whatever you happen to be dealing with at this juncture of your life, even if you do not yet consider yourself a healer. I am here to tell you that *you are* a healer whether you realize it yet or not, and you may have many abilities locked within you that are ready to burst free. Every soul has some special gift that is meant to be shared with the world, and every soul's gift is an absolutely unique expression of that individual. What you have to offer, no one else can give. To this truth, there are no exceptions. Furthermore, these gifts always lead to healing. That is their ultimate purpose.

Spirit can use many channels to extend healing to the people around you. For instance, I use words, both as a speaker and a writer, but my words are just a vehicle that carries a Power far greater than the mere symbols I select. Healing does not actually occur through words. It is the *energy* behind the words that heals. Likewise, a musician's songs may carry the gift of healing to the awareness of listeners; a politician may become a great peacemaker, which the world is desperately in need of now; an artist's paintings may arouse joy and remind lost and struggling souls of the beauty that is possible in life; a business executive's generosity may inspire others in ways no one can predict. These gifts, though, have little to do with the forms through which they are shared. Once again, it is the energy behind them that contains the true healing propensity.

As what might be called a "reluctant healer" myself, in this chapter I'd like to present a few key guidelines to aid new healers in understanding, and accepting, their own role as healers of the world. Whatever your specific gifts turn out to be, a few things remain constant for all healers. This section will also serve as a review of many of the book's healing lessons.

The Healer Inspires the Patient to Choose Life

This one is simple, though it may sound contradictory. Healers do not heal; they *inspire* healing. In the strictest sense, the patient heals him- or herself. The role of the healer is not to heal the patient but to help the patient to choose health. The healer does not salvage the patient from death, but inspires the person to live. This is accomplished through the healer's ability to accept and channel love and the joy of living into the patient's awareness. The healer brings hope and the possibility of happiness into the patient's world, thereby teaching the patient that they deserve and should *want* to live. This can occur through words or actions, or merely through the silent presence of one grounded in the now.

The Healer Must Be Free from Fear

In every circumstance, fear represents a primary obstacle to healing. It is a negative emotion of such intensity that it fully disrupts Source energy from being received. Therefore, releasing this negative emotion represents a major step to overcoming diseases, as well as helping others to do the same. That is why if a healer is to be successful, they must actively work to remain free from the fear-bound state. This is one of the healer's major obligations, and it was my own primary challenge when Jordan was sick.

On the surface, there seem to be many types of fear. There is the fear of death, sickness, and financial ruin; the fear of embarrassment and social rejection; the fear of physical and emotional pain; the fear of failure; and strange as it may sound, the fear of success. Then there are more subtle fears, such as the fear of releasing our need to manipulate and control other people and our circumstances; the fear of trust; the fear of expressing love under the ridiculous guise that it might make us appear weak; the fear of vulnerability, and on and on. Yet, whatever form fear may appear to take, the answer to overcoming it is always the same: the abandonment of personal judgment and the development of trust and faith. What this means is, you must realize that you do not always understand what is best. This is what a lack of judgment really means. You cease attempting to determine what you should do and what you should avoid, realizing that you simply do not know. You then become free to act from the present moment in whatever way feels most natural at the time.

There is a great traditional Eastern story about a Chinese farmer and his son that demonstrates this point wonderfully.

A farmer had just a single horse and an only son to help him tend his crops. One day after a storm destroyed their barn, the farmer's horse escaped and disappeared into the nearby mountains.

The farmer's neighbor came over and expressed his pity to the farmer for his loss. "This is terrible, Farmer," the neighbor cried. "Now what will you do? You have no horse to help you plow your fields."

But the farmer merely shrugged his shoulders indifferently. "Good, bad, who knows?" he replied.

In fact, the next day the horse returned on its own, and the animal was not alone. Twelve wild horses had followed it back to the farmer's property, and he and his son quickly rounded them up.

Hearing about this, the same neighbor came over again. "Amazing luck, Farmer! Now you have thirteen horses to help you with your work!"

Once more, however, the farmer merely shrugged his shoulders. "Good, bad, who knows?" he said.

The next day the farmer's son was trying to tame one of the wild horses when he was thrown from the animal's back. The son landed so hard on the ground that he broke both his legs.

This time the neighbor hurried over, shedding tears of sympathy. "This is terrible, Farmer! It is a tragedy! Now what will you do? Your son has broken both his legs, and you will have to tend your crops all alone. It is too much work for an old man like you."

The farmer shook his head, shrugged his shoulders, and lifted his palms to the sky as if to say, *Good, bad, who knows?*

Within a week following this incident, there was a commotion in the farmer's community when the Chinese army unexpectedly marched into town. Apparently there was a great battle being waged nearby, and while the cause was hopeless, the army was drafting every able-bodied male to come join the fight. They would likely all die, but they would die as heroes.

The farmer's son was spared due to his injured legs.

"Incredible luck!" the neighbor exclaimed over a cup of warm sake later that same night.

"Good, bad, who knows?" answered the farmer.

What is good and what is bad? Do you think you know?

The Healer Must Be Free from Guilt

Guilt, too, plays a key role in keeping us chained to pain and disease. Those who feel guilty automatically feel unworthy, and as a result they cannot accept their true power to heal. First of all, the guilty do not believe they deserve healing. Second, to see yourself as guilty is to separate yourself from your Self, since guilt paints an image in your mind of who and what you are that is antithetical to what and who you are in truth. This discrepancy creates an illusory image of yourself, which is inherently weak and lacking the ability to heal and which disconnects you from Self.

The truth about your soul — and everyone's soul — is that it is fully innocent, perfectly holy, filled with power, and forever invulnerable. So to draw an image in your head and beliefs that is at variance with this fundamental truth, in any way, is to cut your awareness off from your Self and your natural ability to heal. This induces a "split mind" as *A Course in Miracles* refers to it, with your awareness becoming divided between the ego state and your core Self.

This is why the healing of guilt is so crucial to the healing of the body. We cannot fully embrace Truth until we have relinquished all notions of guilt; we cannot know our Self until guilt has been banished from our minds; we cannot heal, or help others to heal, until the barriers against healing have all been undone — not through force, but through gentleness and care.

The Healer Must Cultivate an Awareness of the Present Moment

No matter what your particular contribution to the world's healing turns out to be — even if it seems wholly unrelated to the process of healing as the world sees it — in order to allow Chi to express itself fully through your work, you will need to learn to give from a state of pure presence. If there is one thing I have learned along my own path, it is that, no matter how beautifully composed a sentence happens to be, when it is written from a space of emptiness it will express only emptiness. Yet when words are shared from an awareness of unity and a state of presence, no matter how clumsily delivered, they cannot fail to awaken hearts and inspire.

I suspect the same is true of all special healing roles. Therefore my advice is, above all else, you must seek to master the craft of doing what you do while being thoroughly grounded in the flow of the here and now. Only by working from the present moment can your healing gifts flow through you and into the world. Accessing the present, then, is a necessary skill that every healer must fully master.

The Healer Seeks Unity with the Patient

To be clear, unity between the healer and patient is something that is already present, since unity is the underlying reality of life. Therefore it does not need to be sought or achieved so much as recognized and accepted. It is only individual perception that wavers from the state of unity, and only during its earthly incarnation. Healing, in all forms, is attained through finding a momentary connection with the patient, when all guards have been dropped and all sense of division and differences are allowed to disappear. In this sense healers are really not trying to achieve anything in particular; they are attempting to recognize a reality that is already present, already there, but unrecognized due to being hidden beneath the shattered view of separation that characterizes human perception. For the realization of unity to occur, the healer must release all sense of judgment and focus on the illusory differences that appear to separate the healer from the patient. Even the slightest judgment, or sense of division, will cause the awareness of unity to be swept into oblivion. However, the barest willingness to recognize the undivided state will equally, and forcefully, return the true state of union to awareness. For this to occur, then, the healer must accept that they and the patient are identical.

The Healer Must Accept
That They Are Nothing Special

Like so much of our curriculum, this point may sound counterintuitive at first, but if you consider what the word "special" really means, it makes more sense. Specialness implies superiority and differences, whereas healing specifically relies upon the realization of unity, which must entail equality. All souls are equal. There is no difference. How could there be if life is really one?

During the process of healing, the healer is not giving something special to someone who is viewed as less worthy, less special. Just the opposite. The healer is acknowledging, and actually celebrating, the power that all people share, which is the power to create and heal. Once again, it is not the healer who heals, but the patient who heals him- or herself. By acknowledging the patient's ability to heal, the healer aims to awaken the patient to his or her own latent potential to recover. If the healer feels better, wiser, or more powerful than the patient, the opposite occurs; the healer is denying the patient's strength and his or her greatest hope for recovery by actively reinforcing a sense of separation, weakness, and inequality.

This doesn't mean that the healer is unimportant. It is true that you are nothing special, nor am I — but only in the sense that we are not *different* from one another. Viewed in another way, we are all far beyond any earthly definition of special, being eternal, irreplaceable aspects of Life itself and cocreators of the universe. In this sense, we are more than special; we are descendants of God.

The Healer Must Celebrate the Patient's Free Will

Healing cannot be forced on anyone, and so it is not the function of the healer to overpower the patient's will, even if the patient is being self-destructive. To reiterate an earlier point, true healing stems from gentleness and love, not force of any kind, because it extends the will of Source, which is only love. Once the healer falls out of alignment with the state of love, he or she can no longer effectively channel it. This is not a matter of punishment, but a rudimentary law of metaphysics. This law states:

That which you feel within is that which you extend.

Love begets love; fear begets fear.

The Healing of Jordan Young

If the healer gives in to the urge to force or coerce, the healer becomes removed from the spirit of healing and will not be able to inspire it. This can be a frustrating situation, and it represents a source of a major temptation. Often, at least on the surface, it appears to be a loving gesture to attempt to compel healing on behalf of the patient, but the truth is that even the slightest sense of coercion obliterates the state of union. Acceptance, trust, and faith are the characteristics that lead to healing. Do not allow yourself to be fooled into thinking that any form of loveless bullying can provide a worthy vehicle for the healing energy of love.

The Healer Must Accept
That the Body Is Not the Seat of Life

Finally we come to the consideration that may be the hardest to accept, for all souls who have chosen a physical incarnation must still lay some value on the body. However, it is the learning destiny of all who come here to eventually transcend this misplaced assessment, which actually represents the belief that limitation is freedom, and weakness is strength. It is precisely *because* the body is not the seat of life that it can be so easily healed by what *is* strong and free of limitations. The body itself can never be totally free any more than a fence can, being specifically designed to enclose and limit.

The body is not alive in the way most people think of it. It is not what you are, and not what the patient is. It is merely a vehicle that may be used by what has life and what is life. As long as undue importance is invested in what is essentially lifeless, healing is bound to be stunted because the healer is looking to the lack of power *for* power. The Spirit may use the body as an extension and a tool for its own learning and growth, and to teach others to grow and learn. The potential of your Self remains as limitless as its Creator. By turning away from the fixed preoccupation on the physical, and reconnecting with that which lies beyond it, healing is stimulated on all levels — including the body. This means that in order to heal the body, you must seek to transcend it and recognize that it is not you, and therefore it does not need any healing. It cannot limit or hurt or assault your Self. Your life is not dependent on the body's state. The seat of life exists in a state perfectly sheltered from bodily conditions, at peace and safe beyond time, in eternity.

Which brings us to our final consideration...

When Healing Fails

The body is temporary. This fact has been emphasized for a reason over the course of the book. The acceptance of this idea is a major precept upon which all healing rests, even the healing of the body itself. This is so because bodily awareness restricts perception to a narrow corner of the universe and a tiny swatch of time. It seems to be a prison house, though it is not; it imprisons only the voluntary. As stated, the body is best thought of as a temporary learning device, which is used exclusively while you are enrolled in the Earth School curriculum. Once you accept this idea, you are freed from the fear of letting the body go, and you can then freely rise into the spiritual sphere that surrounds us, beyond the body's boundaries. On the other hand, while the body is emphasized, cherished, and clung to as if your life depends on it, your perspective will necessarily remain restricted to it due to fear.

One thing we must always be mindful of as healers is that sickness is often used as a way to bond with the body in order to deepen the sense of the body's reality and the individual's connection with it. This maneuver is always a response to inner, typically unconscious, fear. Because of this, there will be times when healing will fail, despite the healer's and the patient's efforts to recover. Without the patient's desire to get better, which necessarily suggests they have lost their fear of healing, healing is destined to be stunted. How could it not? The best a healer can do in such a circumstance is to accept healing on behalf of the patient, and recognize that, despite appearances, the patient is not a body any more than the healer is. Even when an illness becomes critical, the patient is not actually in any real danger; death itself is nothing but an appearance of changing forms. What the patient is in reality can never be threatened. It is to this truth the healer must remain faithful.

The Little Swell

There is a lovely parable that likens the journey of awakening to a swell's passage across the ocean. There are various versions of the story, and I would like to share my own with you now.

One clear summer day, a family of ocean swells was traveling across the surface of the sea. The journey was a joyful one, the day was calm and warm, and the swells traveled along without a care, enjoying the journey together.

Then one of the swells began looking into the distance. Up ahead there was an island, and the little swell watched in curiosity as another family of swells raced toward the land. To the little swell's horror, the other swells hit the rocky cliffs that formed the island's shoreline, cresting and breaking in tumultuous explosions of whitewater before disappearing from sight as if they had never even existed.

The little swell became very afraid, and it started screaming. One of the elder swells of the family heard the little swell's cries and asked what was wrong.

"Look!" shouted the little swell. "We're headed for that island! We must change our course or we're all doomed!"

The elder swell peered into the distance and observed what the little swell was referring to. Then it began to laugh.

"Why are you laughing?" asked the little swell in frustration. "Don't you see? We're all going to die!"

"Yes, I see," said the elder swell, "but there is something you seem to have forgotten. You are not just an ordinary swell. *You are* the sea."

Spiritual awakening is a journey of letting go and coming to peace with each stage of your life as it unfolds. This includes the process we call death, though true awakening cannot honestly be called death. People think that when they die, they go to Heaven, but this is really backward; when you die, you come to earth. Heaven is your Home. It is earth that is a land of death, which is why death seems to be all around you while you journey through time. In Heaven, all things last forever, for there are no bodies that age and sicken and die, and the passage of time does not there exist. Heaven is not *endless* time; it is *no time*. Therefore there is also no sickness, no loss, no pain, nor separation. It is truly the land of no parting, for in Heaven you need never say good-bye to those you love. Can the process of leaving this world and returning Home really be considered death, or is it a birth?

The fear of death is gradually relinquished through the recognition that we are not just temporary swells moving across the face of the sea, but the water that makes up the ocean itself. It is the sea that is our true Identity, despite appearances. Our journey through Earth School is the same as the journey of an ocean wave that forgets, for just a tiny flick in its eternal existence, that it is more than just a temporary wave. It is the water of Life.

Our scientists tell us that the universe we live in is actually composed of pure energy, though our eyes do not see it that way. They also tell us that this energy is eternal. It may change in form, but never can it be made to succumb to nothingness. When water is brought to a boil it turns into steam, which rises into the air and seems to vanish into nothingness. Yet the water's journey has not ended because its form has changed and we have lost sight of it.

This is true of your existence as well. When any form seems to die, it has merely shifted into another state of existence. This means that every seeming death must also be a birth into a new state, a fresh experience. Some of these shifts we cannot trace — such as when a person leaves their body — but many are quite clear. One classic example involves the metamorphosis of a caterpillar enwrapped in a cocoon, which grows and develops unseen by the world until it comes time for it to free itself, break its bonds, and emerge as a butterfly. Likewise, the body is also a form of cocoon, and you, too, are a butterfly.

Jordan Lived!

Even after all this time the sun never says to the earth, "You owe me." Look what a love like that can do. It lights up the whole sky.

— HAFIZ

On a cloudless summer morning two months after Jordan started taking Xalkori, Kirsten and I made the three-hour drive to Portland. We followed the same route I had taken the day I hurried to meet Jordan in the intensive care unit at OHSU. Then, I hardly registered the natural beauty that makes this particular highway one of the most scenic drives in the Pacific Northwest, as it crosses the lush green Cascade Mountain Range and angles past majestic, snowcapped Mount Hood — the highest peak in Oregon, which shares a remarkable resemblance to the famous profile of Mount Fuji in Japan.

This time, the journey was different. This time, there was no hurry, no fear. This time we took it all in. And this time, I was not alone.

When we arrived in the City of Roses, we found Jordan at the

Knight Cancer Institute's bone marrow transplant clinic, which is on the fourteenth floor of OHSU Hospital. He was recovering from the bone marrow transplant that ultimately saved his life. After the initial mix up with the Xalkori, the medication finally arrived on the following Monday, just as the company promised it would, and the drug proved to be Jordan's golden ticket to survival. Though we lived in a state of barely subdued panic the whole time, the medication kept Jordan's symptoms in check long enough for the medical team at the Knight Institute to scramble and arrange for the transplant. As it turned out, Jordan only had to wait a little over a month from the time he was eventually released from OHSU to the time he was checking into the transplant center. This must have qualified for some kind of record to prepare for such a complicated procedure, but somehow the remarkable staff at the Knight Institute pulled it off.

The fact that the transplant was able to happen so quickly is a testament to the genuine concern and determination of the medical staff that saw to Jordan's care. A special thank-you goes out to Dr. Maziarz who, once again, led the charge and guided the transplant procedure from start to finish — but the entire team there performed with exemplary professionalism and dedication, which in my view transcended the standard obligations in such situations.

It also helped that a bone marrow donor was rapidly found who proved to be an excellent genetic match for Jordan. This does not always happen, and the selection of a donor is one of the most critical steps of the entire procedure. Get this step wrong and the patient may suffer from life-threatening complications afterward, or the procedure may fail entirely. As it turned out, the donation came from a total stranger. We still do not know why this person chose to bequeath such a personal gift when he did. All we know is that it was another one of the blessings that collided with Jordan's situation at just the right moment.

As of this writing, over three years have passed since the string of co-incidences intervened in Jordan's destiny. I'm happy to report that he is still 100 percent cancer free and doing well. For a while he started taking classes at a local community college, hoping to one day join the United States Forest Service. However, he has since revised his goals. He now wants to work with medical patients who are going through struggles similar to what he survived, though he has yet to determine in what capacity. Jordan still meditates, and he has come to view life as a spiritual journey, not a physical one. He is a remarkably awake person for such a young man, and I believe he will ultimately become a great teacher of healing. He and Brittany are no longer dating, but they are still the best of friends and expect to always be a part of each other's lives. Some experiences are so powerful they transcend the rise and fall of romantic relationships, forming a bond that is destined to last forever. Like life, the form of a relationship may change, but that does not mean it must end.

As for Jordan's family, he has done much mending with his mom, and their relationship has matured significantly, though like all relationships healing is a work in progress. Jordan still lives at home, but his father has moved out, which seems to have reduced the stress and conflict that coincided with Jordan's disease.

While the course of Jordan's illness was terrifying and traumatic for everyone at the time, the book you hold in your hands would not have been possible had he not gone through the experience of journeying to the brink of death and returning with a miracle of hope for all of us to share in and take strength from. I hope it has inspired you, whoever you are. In the end, his journey was as clear a testament to the power of love as any I've personally experienced. I believe that it was love, more than anything else, that saved him. The love of his friends and family; the love of the doctors and nurses and the other medical stars who cared for him; and the love of the man who donated his time, and of his body, to give a gift to a boy he had never met. Take all other things away, and love, if it is pure and present, will find a way because it does one mighty, all-important thing: it awakens the patient to the highest joy of life and convinces them that they deserve to live.

When the patient makes the decision, from the depths of their soul, to recover, and when the conditions of the three Special Principles of Healing are satisfied, all the forces of the universe are ushered to save that person, which is the moment when it can be truly said that *all things become possible* — a medication that had not worked before will suddenly begin working; the right healer will show up at just the right moment; the patient will be in the perfect place at the perfect time; or the patient may simply rise up, cast off their disease, and choose life.

When Jordan first became ill, I could never have imagined that it would lead to this book, which I believe was meant as a gift for you, for me, and for everyone — not just Jordan. The words I spoke to him that day just after I arrived at the ICU, where he lay broken and dying, still ring with truth every time I call them to mind, like a gift sent directly from God, the only true Healer. I'd like to invite you to take these words with you along your own journey, which is likely to be as unique as the prints that mark the tips of your fingers. Be sure to make them your own and share them with everyone you encounter who is struggling with the throes of disease, pain, or fear in any form:

With love, all things can be healed; with love, hope is always justified; with love, nothing is impossible.

Acknowledgments

The saying "it takes a village to raise a child" could just as easily be applied to book writing. So, in one respect, thanks are due to all my family, friends, teachers, and everyone who has participated in educating and making me who I am today. Since I cannot name, nor even recall, them all, I would like to specifically thank a few key individuals who played a role, in one way or another, in "raising" the particular child you are now holding in your hands.

First, my deepest thanks to Jordan Young for the honor of allowing me to share his very personal and profound story with the world. I know it is Jordan's most fervent wish that the pain he endured not go to waste, but be used to ease another's pain; that his journey through the darkness of disease and fear become a light to guide those similarly lost; that his story not be swept away and covered over by the mists of passing time, but preserved as a testament to what becomes possible when a human being chooses life.

And so it is.

Gratitude is also due to the staffs at St. Charles Cancer Center in Bend, Oregon, as well as OHSU Hospital and the Knight Cancer Institute in Portland, especially the intensive care unit and transplant center. Without their care, which went far beyond physical treatments and medications, Jordan could not have survived. In my opinion, it was their driving, emotional support that contributed to Jordan's survival more than any of the medical treatments he received. A special thank-you must certainly be included for Dr. Bill Martin of the St. Charles Cancer Center, who functioned as the primary oncologist in Jordan's treatment, and Dr. Richard Maziarz with the Knight Cancer Institute, who oversaw Jordan's bone marrow transplant and ferociously fought to save Jordan's life when he fell from the sky and landed in OHSU's ICU, in the immediate process of dying.

Thanks as well to the staff at New World Library, one of world's great publishers of life-changing books, and a real force for spiritual growth and hope in a world that is far too often dedicated to violence and riddled with suffering. Ushering light into the darkness is their primary mission, and for that they deserve gratitude beyond words. I'd like to especially thank Georgia Hughes, the editorial director of New World Library, who read through a draft of the book and offered valuable suggestions and encouragement.

Jeff Campbell edited the book and did an amazing job at guiding me through cutting out the weak parts, filling in the missing blanks, and expanding on the book's strengths. Thank you, Jeff!

Finally, my wife, Kirsten, emotionally supported me during Jordan's disease, and financially supported me (to a great extent, anyway), while I wrote this book. Without her, this child might never have been born, much less raised. I love you, Baby Doll, and I will forever be grateful that you have become a part of my life. You and I, we go together...

Principles of Healing and Special Principles of Healing

Seven Principles of Healing

Principle of Healing 1: All diseases — no matter their form — must be treated at the deepest level in order for the condition to be healed.

Principle of Healing 2: Every thought has an effect on the body.

Principle of Healing 3: Fear thoughts feed disease.

Principle of Healing 4: Love thoughts heal.

Principle of Healing 5: You are a natural-born creator.

Principle of Healing 6: Healing cannot be forced on the patient. It must be actively invited and openly received.

Principle of Healing 7: Total healing can occur only through entering the healing dimension, which is a state of direct union with Source.

Three Special Principles of Healing

Special Principle of Healing 1: The patient must believe healing is possible.

Special Principle of Healing 2: The patient must want to heal.

Special Principle of Healing 3: The patient must feel they deserve to heal.

Endnotes

Page 8: *"Mind doesn't dominate body, it becomes body"*: Candace B. Pert, *Molecules of Emotion: The Science Behind Mind-Body Medicine* (New York: Simon & Schuster, 1999), 187.

Page 65: *Our life is shaped by our mind:* Eknath Easwaran, trans., *The Dhammapada* (Tomales, CA: Nilgiri Press, 2007), 105.

Page 76: *"Sickness is not an accident....[It] is a decision."*: A Course in Miracles: Workbook for Students* (Mill Valley, CA: Foundation for Inner Peace, 2008), 258.

Page 115: *Buddha instructed his followers, "Guard your thoughts, words, and deeds"*: Eknath Easwaran, trans., *The Dhammapada* (Tomales, CA: Nilgiri Press, 2007), 206.

Page 123: *Who is the physician? Only the mind: A Course in Miracles: Manual for Teachers* (Mill Valley, CA: Foundation for Inner Peace, 2008), 18.

Page 144: *For instance, one study performed by the Benson-Henry Institute:* Jeffery A. Dusek et al., "Genomic Counter-Stress Changes Induced by the Relaxation Response," *PLoS ONE* 3, no. 7, e2576 (July 2008), doi:10.1371/journal.pone.0002576, http://journals.plos.org/plosone/article?id=10.1371/journal.pone.0002576.

Page 144: *Another study conducted by UCLA researchers found that certain:* University of California, Los Angeles, "Meditation May Increase Gray Matter," Science Daily, May 13, 2009, http://www.sciencedaily.com/releases/2009/05/090512134655.htm (accessed May 25, 2011).

Page 208: *"This is Palm Sunday, the celebration of the victory": A Course in Miracles: Text* (Mill Valley, CA: Foundation for Inner Peace, 2008), 425.

Recommended Reading

*I*n *The Healing of Jordan Young*, I have stuck almost entirely to spiritual suggestions for treating disease, but there are a variety of interesting natural paths one might utilize to enhance health and healing. My list of recommended reading therefore includes a mix of important topics — from spirituality and meditation to exercise and cookbooks — that both students of awakening and persons concerned with their health may find useful. There is substantial emerging evidence that our diet plays an enormous role in the causation of many so-called Western diseases, such as cancer and heart disease, and exercise has an obvious, direct impact on the condition of the body. For those looking for information on how food impacts health, *The China Study* by Colin T. Campbell and Thomas M. Campbell is a must read. If you are interested in alternative medical therapies, I suggest *The Comprehensive Report on the Cannabis Extract Movement and the Use of Cannabis Extracts to Treat Diseases* by Justin Kander and Nicholas Davey. This is the only self-published book on the list, and it is not what you would call an "entertaining" read. However, it does a good job of documenting the startling discovery that cannabis oil, which is not to be confused with medical marijuana, holds astounding anticancer properties.

A Course in Miracles. Mill Valley, CA: Foundation for Inner Peace, 2008.

Aggrawal, Bharat, and Debora Yost. *Healing Spices: How to Use 50 Everyday and Exotic Spices to Boost Health and Beat Disease*. New York: Sterling Publishing, 2011.

Balch, Phyllis A. *Prescription for Nutritional Healing: A Practical A-to-Z Reference to Drug Free Remedies Using Vitamins, Minerals, Herbs & Food Supplements*. 5th ed. Garden City, NY: Avery Trade, 2010.

Bittman, Mark. *How to Cook Everything Vegetarian: 2000 Simple Recipes for Great Food*. Boston: Houghton Mifflin Harcourt, 2006.

Blake, Tobin. *Everyday Meditation: 100 Daily Meditations for Health, Stress Relief, and Everyday Joy*. Novato, CA: New World Library, 2012.

Campbell, Adam. *The Women's Health Big Book of Exercises: Four Weeks to a Leaner, Sexier, Healthier YOU!* New York: Rodale Books, 2009.

Campbell, T. Colin, and Thomas M. Campbell II. *The China Study: The Most Comprehensive Study of Nutrition Ever Conducted and the Startling Implications for Diet, Weight Loss, and Long Term Health*. Dallas: BenBella Books, 2006.

Kander, Justin, and Nicholas Davey. *The Comprehensive Report on the Cannabis Extract Movement and the Use of Cannabis Extracts to Treat Diseases*. Amazon Digital Services, 2013.

Moscowitz, Isa Chandra, and Terry Hope Romero. *Veganomigon: The Ultimate Vegan Cookbook*. Cambridge, MA: Da Capo Lifelong Books, 2007.

Pert, Candace B. *Molecules of Emotion: The Science Behind Mind Body Medicine*. New York: Simon & Schuster, 1999.

Siegel, Bernie S. *The Art of Healing: Uncovering Your Inner Wisdom and Potential for Self-Healing*. Novato, CA: New World Library, 2013.

————. *Love, Medicine & Miracles: Lessons Learned about Self-Healing from a Surgeon's Experience with Exceptional Patients*. New York: Harper & Row, 1986; reprint, New York: William Morrow, 1998.

Stone, Gene. *Forks Over Knives: The Plant-Based Way to Health*. New York: The Experiment, 2011.

Tolle, Eckhart. *The Power of Now: A Guide to Spiritual Enlightenment*. Novato, CA: New World Library, 2004.

Villepigue, James, and Hugo Rivera. *The Body Sculpting Bible for Men: The Way to Physical Perfection*. New York: Hatherleigh Press, 2011.

Weil, Andrew. *Spontaneous Healing: How to Discover and Embrace Your Body's Natural Ability to Maintain and Heal Itself*. New York: Ballantine Books, 2000.

About the Author

Tobin Blake is the author of *Everyday Meditation: 100 Daily Meditations for Health, Stress Relief, and Everyday Joy,* which was selected as one of the best books of 2012 by *Conversations Magazine;* and *The Power of Stillness: Learn Meditation in 30 Days,* an alternate selection of *One Spirit Book Club.* Since the publication of his first book, Tobin has appeared on numerous radio and television shows, and he has held workshops on meditation, mind-body healing, and spiritual awakening.

Tobin has studied various spiritual traditions and has been meditating for over two decades. He received his formal training in meditation through Self-Realization Fellowship, an international organization founded by Paramahansa Yogananda, and he is also a longtime student of *A Course in Miracles.*

Born and raised in Los Angeles, Tobin now resides in Bend, Oregon, a high-desert community on the eastern flank of the Cascade Mountains of central Oregon — a varied land of rivers, temperate rain forests, and frosted mountain peaks. He has two daughters, and when he isn't writing or teaching meditation, he enjoys hiking, camping, and various other outdoor activities, as well as sampling Oregon's delightful pinot noirs. For information about the author and his work, please visit his website at www.TobinBlake.com, or connect with him on Facebook at www.Facebook.com/TobinBlake.

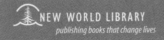